Keto Diet Guide For Beginners

Your Complete and Definitive Guide to losing
weight you will learn how to follow the
Ketogenic diet even if you are a
beginners getting back
in shape!

I0421634

Written by Mark Sell

TABLE OF CONTENTS

INTRODUCTION

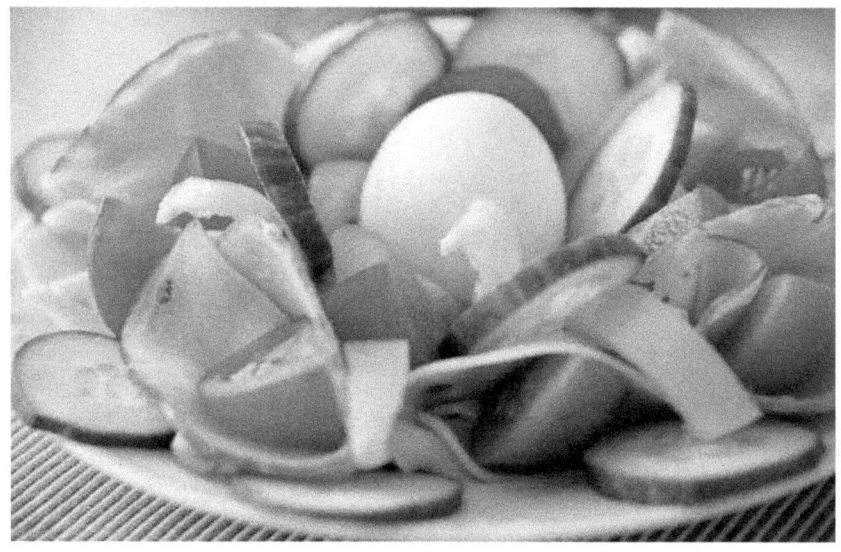

A keto diet is well known for being an low carb diet, where the body produces ketones in the liver to be used as energy. It's referred to as many different names ketogenic diet, low carb diet, low carb high fat (LCHF), etc.

When you eat something high in carbs, your body will produce glucose and insulin.

Glucose is the easiest molecule for your body to convert and use as energy so that it will be chosen over any other energy source.

Insulin is produced to process the glucose in your bloodstream by taking it around the body.

Since the glucose is being used as a primary energy, your fats are not needed and are therefore stored. Typically on an normal, higher carbohydrate diet, the body will use glucose as the main form of energy. By lowering the intake of carbs, the body is induced into a state known as ketosis.

Ketosis is a natural process the body initiates to help us survive when food intake is low. During this state, we produce ketones, which are produced from the breakdown of fats in the liver.

The end goal of a properly maintained keto diet is to force your body into this metabolic state. We don't do this through starvation of calories but starvation of carbohydrates. Reading this Guide will enlight you on the keto diet, stay cool!!

Ketogenic diets are basically designed to induce a state of ketosis in the body. When the amount of glucose in the body becomes too low, the body switches to fat as an alternative source of energy.

The body has two primary fuel sources which are:

Fat deposits are stored in the form of triglycerides. They are normally broken down into long-chain fatty acids and glycerol. Stripping off the glycerol from the triglyceride molecule allows for the release of the three free fatty acid (FFA) molecules into the bloodstream to be used as energy.

The glycerol molecule goes into the liver where three molecules of it combine to form one glucose molecule. Therefore, as your body burns fat, it also produces glucose as a by-product. This glucose can be used to fuel parts of the brain as well as other parts of the body that cannot run on FFA.

However, while glucose can travel through the bloodstream on its own, cholesterol and triglycerides need a carrier to move around in the bloodstream. Cholesterol and triglycerides are packaged in a carrier called low-density lipoprotein, or LDL. Thus, the larger the LDL particle, the more triglycerides it contains.

The overall process of burning fat deposits for energy produces carbon dioxide, water, and compounds called ketones.

Ketones are produced by the liver from free fatty acids. There are composed of 2 groups of atoms linked together by a carbonyl functional group.

The body has no capability to store ketones and therefore they must be either used or excreted. The body excrete them either through the breath as acetone or through the urine as acetoacetate.

Ketones can be used by body cells as a source of energy. Also, the brain can make use of ketones in generating about 70-75% of its energy requirement.

Like alcohol, ketones take priority as a fuel source over carbohydrates. This implies that when they are high in the bloodstream, they must be burned first before glucose can be used as a fuel.

What Causes Ketosis

When you start eating less amounts of carbohydrates, your body gets smaller supply of glucose to use as energy compared to before.

The decrease in the amount of consumed carbohydrates and the subsequent reduction in the amount of available glucose, slowly forces the body to move into the state of ketosis. Thus, the body goes into a state of ketosis when there is not enough amount of glucose available to the body cells.

Starvation Induced Ketosis

Fasting and starvation states usually involve reduced or no intake of food that the body can digest and convert into glucose. While starvation is involuntary, fasting is a more conscious choice you make to intentionally not eat.

However, the body enters into a "starvation mode" whenever you are sleeping, when you skip a meal or when you intentionally go on a fast. The lack of food intake results in a reduction in blood glucose levels. As a result, the body starts to break down it glycogen (stored glucose) stores for energy.

The glycogen is converted back into glucose and used as energy by the body. In this state, the body also starts to burn its stored fats. Thus, the production of ketone bodies (ketogenesis) is induced by a lack of available glucose.

Any time the amount of ketones in the blood outnumber the molecules of glucose, the body cells will start making use of the ketones as their source of energy.

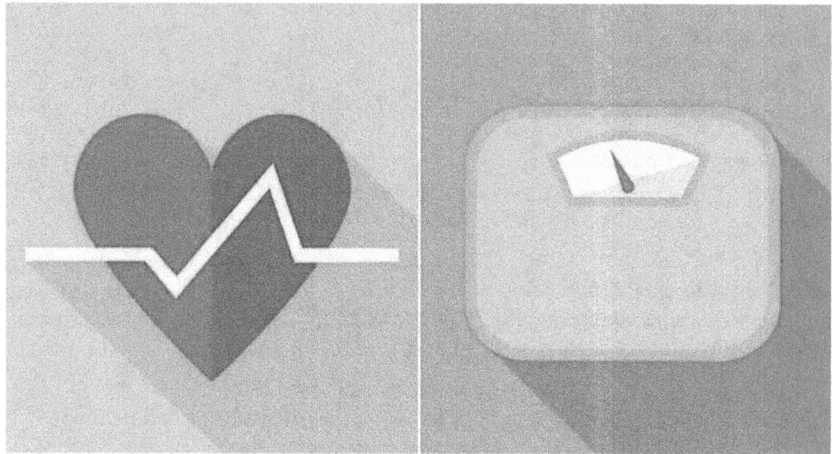

When you eat a diet rich in carbohydrates, your body converts those carbs into glucose (blood sugar). Since carbohydrates are turned into sugar, your blood sugar levels rise.

When blood sugar levels rise, it signals your body to create insulin, which carries glucose to your cells to be used for energy.

Glucose is the preferred energy source of your body. As long as you keep eating carbohydrates, your body will keep turning it into sugar, thereby burning that sugar for energy. In other words, when glucose is present, your body will refuse to burn off its fat stores.

Since carbs are your body's preferred energy source, the only way to start burning fat is by removing carbs.

Cutting carbs depletes your glycogen stores (stored glucose). And with no glucose available for energy, your body has no choice but to start burning its fat stores. Your body starts converting fatty acids into ketones, a metabolic state known as ketosis, and the basis of a ketogenic diet.

What Are Ketones?

In ketosis, your liver converts fatty acids into ketone bodies or ketones. These byproducts become your body's new energy source. When you increase your fat intake, your body responds by becoming "keto-adaptive," or more efficient at burning fat.

Ketosis is a natural survival function of your body. It helps your body function on stored body fat when food is not readily available. Similarly, the keto diet focuses on "starving" your body of carbohydrates, transforming your body into an fat-burning state and supplementing with optimal nutrition.

The three main ketone bodies that your metabolism produces are:

Acetoacetate (AcAc)

Beta-hydroxybutyric acid (BHB)

Acetone

The Difference Between Keto, Low-Carb, and Atkins

Too often, the keto diet gets lumped in with other low-carbohydrate diets, like the Atkins Diet. There are an few key differences between them.

Difference In Carbohydrate Intake

The main difference between keto and low-carb is the macronutrient levels. Low-carb diets are considered any diet with a carb intake under about 100-150 grams of carbs per day. It's likely that you'll have to lower your carb intake much more to enter a state of ketosis.

The Atkins Diet is different from keto because of its different phases, which range from severely restricting carbs to adding a liberal amount of carbs (about 80-100 grams daily) back into the diet.

The keto diet works best when you stick to consistently low carb intake under about 50 grams per day for most people.

Difference In Protein Intake

Most low-carb diets are also high-protein diets. However, the keto diet ranges in protein intake, from moderate (around 20% of your total calories) to high-protein intake.

High-protein intake was once thought to spike blood sugar on a ketogenic diet, but there's evidence that you don't need to worry about gluconeogenesis as much as once thought. Still, diets like Atkins depend heavily on protein, without healthy, low-carb veggies for a majority of the diet.

If you're unsure of your optimal protein intake, check out the Keto Calculator to get your unique macronutrient guidelines.

Difference In Goals

The goals between these diets vary as well. The goal of keto is to enter ketosis, weaning your body off burning glucose for fuel for the long-term.

You may never enter ketosis with a low-carb diet. And although you may enter ketosis for a brief period on the Atkins Diet, you'll pop right back out in Phases 3 and 4 as you reintroduce higher levels of carbohydrate-rich foods.

Ketogenic Diet Macronutrients

Macronutrients seem to be the cornerstone of any keto diet, but contrary to popular opinion, there is no ONE macronutrient ratio that works for everyone.

Instead, you're going to have a completely different set of macros than your friend or your mother based on:

Your physical and mental goals

Your health history

Your activity level

The best way to figure these numbers out quickly is to refer to this macronutrient calculator.

Outside of your personal macros, there are general macro guidelines for a ketogenic diet:

70-80% of calories from fats

20-25% of calories from protein

5-10% of calories from carbohydrates

Below, these percentages are broken down into grams. Remember, these should be used as a guideline only. Your macronutrient goals will vary depending on your particular lifestyle.

Fat Intake

Fat is known as the cornerstone of the keto diet because fat does not raise your blood glucose like protein and carbs.

It was once thought that, in order to get into ketosis, you needed to eat massive amounts of fat on a daily basis. However, that's just not true.

The real secret to getting into ketosis is to cut carbs. You can modulate your fat intake from there. However, the accepted rule of thumb for most keto dieters is to stick to anywhere from 70-80% of your calories from healthy fats.

That means, if you're consuming 2,000 calories per day, you would need 144 to 177 grams of fat.

Protein Intake

Protein has gotten a bad rap in the keto community. Some experts claimed that eating too much protein on a very low-carb diet could trigger an metabolic effect called gluconeogenesis.

Protein is extremely important on the keto diet especially if you're active or an athlete.

Ideally, you should consume at least 0.8 grams of protein per pound of lean body mass to prevent muscle loss. For those of you with a extremely active lifestyle, 1 gram of protein per pound of lean body mass is ideal.

To calculate your lean body mass, you have to:

Calculate your body fat percentage. Click here to read how.

Subtract your body fat % from 100%. This will be your lean body mass %.

Multiply your lean body mass % by your total weight.

Or, you can check out the Keto Calculator to figure out your ideal protein intake.

So while most keto sites recommend 10-15% of total calories from protein, know that you can eat an lot more without raising your blood glucose or kicking you out of ketosis.

Carbohydrate Intake

Most people who want to get into ketosis should get about 5-10% of total calories from carbohydrates.

This usually looks like anywhere from 100-200 calories from carbs or about 25-50 grams of carbohydrates per day.

Most people consume roughly 30 grams of carbohydrates on the keto diet. Depending upon your activity level and health needs, you might be able to consume 80 grams of carbs and remain in ketosis.

Different Types of Ketogenic Diets

There are five main approaches to the ketogenic diet. When deciding which method works best for you, take into account your goals, fitness level, and what's realistic for your lifestyle.

The Standard Ketogenic Diet (SKD)

This is the most common and recommended version of the diet. Here, you stay within 20-50 grams of net carbs per day, focusing on moderate protein intake and high fat intake.

Targeted Ketogenic Diet (TKD)

If you are an active individual, this approach might work best for you. Targeted keto involves eating roughly 25-50 grams of net carbs or less 30 minutes to an hour before exercise.

Cyclical Ketogenic Diet (CKD)

If keto seems intimidating to you, this is an excellent method to start with. You cycle between periods of eating an low-carb diet for several days, followed by a period of eating higher amounts of carbs (typically lasting several days).

High-Protein Ketogenic Diet (HPKD)

This approach is very similar to the standard (SKD) approach. The primary difference is your protein intake. While a standard keto diet will include moderate protein, here you up your protein intake considerably.

Plant-Based Keto

Plant-based keto could range from eating more low-carb vegetables to going keto as a full-on vegan or vegetarian. You can follow the ketogenic diet as a vegetarian or as a vegan, but it will take a lot of work and effort to do this safely.

What Can You Eat on a Keto Diet?

Now that you understand the basics behind the keto diet, it's time to hit the grocery store.

On the keto diet, you'll enjoy nutrient-dense foods including meat, vegetables, nuts and seeds, and plenty of healthy fats.

You'll also avoid grains, legumes, processed foods, and most fruits. Consume these keto-friendly foods while staying within your macro guidelines:

Meat, Eggs, And Nuts

All meat and seafood are included on the keto diet, as long as they're, not breaded or fried.

Always choose the highest quality meat, you can afford, selecting grass-fed and organic beef whenever possible, wild-caught fish, and pasture-raised poultry, pork, and eggs.

Nuts and seeds are also fine and best eaten raw (not roasted or coated in sugar).

Enjoy:

Beef, preferably fattier cuts like steak, veal, roast, ground beef and stews

Poultry, including chicken breasts, quail, duck, turkey and wild game try to focus on the darker, fattier meats

Pork, including pork loin, tenderloin, chops, ham, and sugar-free bacon

Fish, including mackerel, tuna, salmon, trout, halibut, cod, catfish, and mahi-mahi

Shellfish, including oysters, clams, crab, mussels, and lobster

Organ meats, including heart, liver, tongue, kidney, and offal

Eggs, including deviled, fried, scrambled and boiled use the whole egg

Lamb

Goat

Vegetarian sources, like macadamia nuts, almonds, and nut butter

Low-Carb Vegetables

On a keto meal plan, feel free to fill your plate with low-carb vegetables.

Vegetables are a great way to get a healthy dose of micronutrients, thus preventing vitamin deficiencies on keto.

Enjoy low-carb vegetables like leafy greens, and cruciferous veggies, aiming to eat veggies that contain fewer than 5 grams of net carbs per serving.

Enjoy these low carb vegetables:

Leafy greens, such as kale, spinach, swiss chard and arugula

Cruciferous vegetables, including cabbage, cauliflower, and zucchini

Lettuces, including iceberg, romaine, and butterhead

Fermented vegetables like sauerkraut and kimchi

Other vegetables such as mushrooms, asparagus, and celery

Keto-Friendly Dairy

If you can tolerate dairy, it is allowed on the keto diet. Choose the highest quality you can reasonably afford, selecting grass-fed, whole-fat, and organic dairy whenever possible.

Keto-friendly dairy options include:

Butter and ghee

Heavy cream and heavy whipping cream

Fermented dairy products like yogurts and kefir

Sour cream

Hard and soft cheeses

Low-Sugar Fruits

Approach fruit with caution on keto, as it contains high amounts of sugar and carbohydrates. If you are craving something light and sweet, grab a handful of berries, such as blueberries or raspberries, as a treat.

Enjoy these low sugar fruits:

Avocadoes (the one fruit you can enjoy in abundance)

Organic berries, such as raspberries, blueberries, strawberries, and cranberries

Healthy Fats And Oils

You can enjoy both animal fats (saturated fats) and plant-based fats on a healthy keto diet.

Healthy fat sources include grass-fed butter, tallow, and ghee or coconut oil, olive oil, sustainable palm oil and MCT oil from plants.

Enjoy these fats and oils on keto:

Butter and ghee

Lard

Mayonnaise

Coconut oil, coconut butter

Flaxseed oil

Olive oil

Sesame seed oil

MCT oil and MCT powder

Walnut oil

Olive oil, avocado oil

Herbs And Spices

Use seasonings freely on keto just make sure they don't have any added sugar.

To add flavor to dishes, consider purchasing fresh herbs at the store.

Pro tip: If you store fresh herbs in an mason jar filled with water in the fridge, they will last up to two weeks.

Foods to Avoid on a Keto Diet

It's best to avoid the following foods on a keto diet due to their high carb content.

When starting keto, do a purge of your fridge and cupboards. Donate any unopened items and throw the rest away.

Grains

Grains are loaded with carbs, so it's best to avoid all grains on keto. Whole grains, wheat, pasta, rice, oats, barley, rye, corn, and quinoa are all out. Instead, try one of these substitutes.

Beans And Legumes

While many vegans and vegetarians rely beans for their protein content, they are actually incredibly high-carb. Avoid eating kidney beans, chickpeas, black beans, and lentils.

Higher-Sugar Fruits

While many fruits are packed with antioxidants and other micronutrients, they're also high in fructose, which will kick you out of ketosis.

Avoid apples, mangos, pineapple and other fruits (with the exception of small amounts of berries).

Starchy Veggies

Avoid starchy vegetables like potatoes, sweet potatoes, some squash, parsnips, and carrots.

Like fruit, there are health benefits to these foods. However, you can find those vitamins and minerals from low-carb sources ones that won't kick you out of ketosis.

Sugar

This includes, but is not limited to desserts, artificial sweeteners, smoothies, soda, and fruit juice.

Even condiments like ketchup and BBQ sauce are usually filled with sugar, so put down the ketchup bottle. If you are craving a dessert, try one of these keto-friendly recipes instead.

Alcohol

Some alcoholic beverages are low-glycemic and appropriate for a ketogenic diet. However, keep in mind that when you drink alcohol, your liver will preferentially process the ethynol and stop producing ketones.

If you're on a ketogenic diet to lose weight, keep your alcohol consumption to a minimum. If you're craving a cocktail, stick to low-sugar mixers and avoid most beer and wine.

Seed Oils

Seed oils are heavily processed and can become oxidized (aka, rancid) when you heat them. Avoid corn oil, canola oil, peanut oil, and grapeseed oil. They also contain large amounts of omega–6 fatty acids, which are inflammatory in large amounts.

Health Benefits of a Keto Diet

A ketogenic diet has been associated with incredible health benefits that stretch way beyond weight loss. Here are just an few ways keto may help you feel better, stronger, and more clear-headed:

Keto For Weight Loss

Probably what the keto diet is most famous for: sustainable fat loss. Keto can significantly decrease body weight, body fat, and body mass while maintaining muscle mass. Keto can also increase fat metabolism during exercise, making it an excellent part of your active lifestyle.

Keto For Endurance Levels

The ketogenic diet may help improve endurance levels for athletes. However, it may take time for athletes to adjust to burning fat instead of glucose for energy.

Keto For Gut Health

Several studies have shown a link between low sugar intake and improvement in symptoms of irritable bowel syndrome (IBS). In fact, one study showed that eating a ketogenic diet can improve abdominal pain and overall quality of life in those with IBS.

Keto For Diabetes

The ketogenic diet helps to balance blood sugar and insulin levels, which helps immensely with metabolic diseases like type 2 diabetes.

Keto For Heart Health

The keto diet can help reduce risk factors for heart disease, including improvement in HDL cholesterol, triglycerides, and LDL cholesterol (related to plaque in the arteries).

Keto For Brain Health

The keto diet may support those with Parkinson's, Alzheimer's disease, and other degenerative brain diseases This is likely because ketone bodies having possible neuroprotective and anti-inflammatory benefits.

Keto For Skin Health

Because ketones and lower blood sugar contribute to overall hormone balance and lower inflammatory markers, the keto diet may be good for skin health. One study suggests that decreased skin inflammation can decrease acne and other skin lesions.

Keto For Epilepsy

The ketogenic diet was created in the early 20th century to help prevent seizures in epileptic patients, especially children. To this day, ketosis is a go-to therapeutic diet for those who suffer from epilepsy.

Keto For Cancer Support

There's a growing body of research that suggests a strict keto diet can help slow tumor growth. Although no one diet can cure or prevent cancer, an low-carb, zero-sugar diet is a great place to start.

Keto For Pms

A estimated 90% of women experience one or more of symptoms associated with PMS. A keto diet can help balance blood sugar, combat chronic inflammation, boost your nutrient stores, and crush cravings all of which may help alleviate your PMS symptoms.

How to Know When You're in Ketosis

You can follow the above macronutrient guidelines, eat the prescribed keto diet foods and avoid grains, starches, and legumes and still struggle to enter ketosis.

Why? Because ketosis is an metabolic state, and you may need to tweak your meal plan, exercise regimen, and other lifestyle choices in order to enter it.

There are plenty of signs and symptoms to suggest you're in ketosis, including:

Weight loss

Fewer cravings

Better mental clarity

More stable energy

But there's only one reliable way to know whether or, not you're in ketosis: Test your ketone levels.

There are three ways to do this:

In your urine with a urine strip

In your blood with a glucose meter

On your breath with a breath meter

The Ketogenic Diet Heirarchy of Needs Testing

Each method has its advantages and disadvantages, with a blood test being the most accurate (but most expensive). Although it's the most affordable, urine testing is typically the least accurate method.

Supplements to Support a Keto Diet

Supplements are a popular way to maximize the benefits of a ketogenic diet. You can't get all of your nutrients from supplements and expect to feel good, but they can help.

Add in these supplements alongside a healthy, whole-food based keto diet for the best results.

Exogenous Ketones

"Exogenous ketones" are supplemental ketones usually beta-hydroxybutyrate or acetoacetate that help kick you into ketosis and give you the energy you need to thrive. You can take exogenous ketones in between meals or for a quick burst of energy before a workout.

MCT Oil And Powder

MCTs (or medium-chain triglycerides) are a type of fatty acid that your body can convert to energy quickly and efficiently. Benefits includes weight loss and energy, among other things. MCTs come from coconuts and are sold mostly in liquid form. Perfect Keto sells them as a delicious and easy-to-use powder.

Collagen Protein

Collagen is the most abundant protein in your body, accounting for about 25-35%. It's the glue that holds your body together as it supports the growth of joints, organs, hair, and connective tissues. Amino acids from collagen supplements may also help with energy production, DNA repair, detox, and healthy digestion.

Micronutrient Supplements

It's tough to get all the micronutrients you need from diet alone regardless of what nutrition regimen you're on. Keto Micro Greens is the solution to getting all your micronutrients in one convenient scoop.

Ketogenic Pre-Workout Supplements

Keto pre-workout supplements like Perfect Keto Perform Pre-Workout can boost physical and cognitive performance without the caffeine crash. It contains exogenous ketones and MCT oil powder for energy, creatine for protein metabolism, branched-chain amino acids for muscle growth and repair, and more.

Whey Protein

One of the best-studied supplements for weight loss support, muscle gain and maintenance, and recovery. Make is sure to choose grass-fed whey only and avoid powders with sugar or any other additives that could spike blood sugar.

Electrolytes

Electrolyte balance is one of the most critical yet most overlooked components of a successful ketogenic diet experience. Especially when you're just starting out. A keto diet can make you excrete more electrolytes than usual so you have to replenish them yourself. Add more sodium, potassium, and calcium to your diet or grab a supplement that can help.

Krill Oil

Get even more of the benefits of an anti-inflammatory keto diet with some high-quality omega-3 fatty acids. Krill oil is just as potent as fish oil, without the fishy aftertaste. Krill also contains phospholipids and a potent antioxidant called astaxanthin that fish oil doesn't.

Blood Sugar Support

Think about adding vitamins, minerals, and herbs to support normal digestion, metabolism, hormone function, and energy production. Take these with higher carb meals to support healthy carbohydrate metabolism or just to promote healthy nutrient absorption.

Is the Ketogenic Diet Safe?

Ketosis is a perfectly safe and natural metabolic state, but it is often confused with a highly dangerous metabolic state called ketoacidosis.

Having ketone levels in the 0.5-5.0mmol/L range is not dangerous, but other risks include a range of issues, from harmless keto flu symptoms to diabetic ketoacidosis, which is not a problem unless you're diabetic.

Ketoacidosis

Diabetic ketoacidosis (DKA) is a dangerous metabolic state that is most commonly seen in people with type 1 diabetes and sometimes type 2 diabetics if they aren't properly managing their insulin and diet.

Keto Flu Symptoms

Many people deal with common side effects similar to flu-like symptoms as they become fat adapted after decades of running on carbs. These temporary symptoms are byproducts of dehydration and low carbohydrate levels while your body adjusts:

Headaches

Lethargy

Nausea

Brain fog

Stomach pain

Low motivation

The keto flu can often be shortened or avoided completely by taking one of our ketone supplements, which help switch the body into ketosis instantly. They make the transition period much shorter and easier.

Different Types of Ketogenic Diets

Over the past several years, people have found different ways to approach the ketogenic diet.

Depending on your goals and fitness level, you may find one type of keto diet fits your lifestyle better than others. No matter which one you choose, the goal should be to shift your body from using carbs to using fat as your primary source of fuel.

Here's a breakdown of the different type of keto diets:

Standard Ketogenic Diet (SKD)

This is the most straightforward approach to the ketogenic diet. On the SKD, you're keeping your total carbs extremely low while focusing most of your macronutrient intake on fat and protein. The goal of SKD is to get into and maintain a state of ketosis, burning fat as your primary source of fuel.

Cyclical Ketogenic Diet (CKD)

The cyclical ketogenic diet is a good choice if your goal is to increase muscle strength and improve exercise performance. When following the CKD you're cycling days of ketosis with days of higher carb intake. A typical CKD will be five to six days eating a keto diet (very low-carb), with one or two days of higher carb intake.

The purpose is to reap the benefits of keto during the days on, and on the re-feeding carb days to restore your glycogen stores for huge amounts of activity.

As mentioned earlier, glucose from carbs is a very readily available source of fuel. For athletes and bodybuilders, this can be a great way to get the best of both worlds.

Targeted Ketogenic Diet(TKD)

The TKD is similar to the standard ketogenic diet, with the exception that you can eat carbohydrates around (before or after) heavy workouts. This approach is for you if you're performing high-intensity workouts for extended periods of time.

If you exercise regularly and are burning fuel at a significant rate, this may be a good strategy for you. Especially if you find yourself "bonking" during workouts when you're in ketosis.

Some athletes notice a decrease in stamina after they've switched to keto.

This approach allows them to benefit from the rapid fuel source of glucose, while also burning it up quickly enough to get back into a ketogenic state. This strategy is best for people who are working out for an hour or more at an moderate to high intensity.

High-Protein Ketogenic Diet

The high-protein keto diet is becoming popular as more people are discovering that they can eat higher protein while still maintaining a ketogenic state.

A high-protein ketogenic diet should be around 30-35% protein, with 60% fat, keeping carbs just as low as you would on a standard ketogenic diet.

This is a good option for people who are active and want to maintain muscle mass. It's also an approach to play with if you're having a hard time sticking to a very high-fat, low- to moderate-protein diet.

Regardless of your macronutrient ratio, the goal is to maintain a ketogenic state for as much of the time as possible, so you can reap all the benefits of being in a ketogenic state.

Benefits of a Keto Diet

Many anecdotal accounts of the keto diet claim rapid weight loss, better brain function, and fewer food cravings. But there are plenty of scientifically-backed benefits of the keto diet as well. Here are just a few:

Blood Sugar Control

Studies have found that people with type 2 diabetes do exceptionally well on a ketogenic diet. Studies show that the extreme reduction in carbs showed an increase in blood glucose control as well as a reduced need for insulin controlling medication.

Fat Loss

Despite higher caloric intake, the ketogenic diet is superior to an low-fat diet for fat loss. Fat loss around the midsection (metabolically active fat) seems to be a specific target in ketogenic fat loss.

Mental Clarity

Many people report feeling enhanced mental sharpness and clarity when following a ketogenic diet. Part of this response may come from higher energy utilization along with the anti-inflammatory effect of the ketogenic diet.

Blood Lipid Profile

Following a ketogenic diet can improve your blood lipid profile. Specifically, it can increase HDL (good cholesterol) and also increase the size of your LDL particles. Larger, fluffier LDL particles are safer because they are less likely to contribute to plaques.

Lower Inflammation

One of the three ketone bodies, beta-hydroxybutyrate (BHB), has been shown to decrease inflammation in your body by blocking an inflammatory signaling pathway.

Heart Disease

Due to its positive effect on both blood lipids and inflammation, the ketogenic diet may benefit those with or at risk for heart disease.

Neurological Disease

The ketogenic diet has been used for over 80 years to treat epilepsy, a disorder in which the nerve cell activity in your brain is disturbed, leading to seizures.

WEEK 1:

MONDAY

Breakfast: Cheesy Keto Bagels

Lunch: Zesty Chili Lime Keto Tuna Salad

Dinner: Nutritious Baked Pork Chops

TUESDAY

Breakfast: Avocado Egg Bowls

Lunch: Low-Carb Romanesco with Cabbage Noodles

Dinner: One-Pan Cheesy Broccoli Chicken Casserole

WEDNESDAY

Breakfast: Breakfast Casserole with Bacon, Egg, and Cheese

Lunch: Grass-Fed Keto Beef Bulgogi

Dinner: Lemon Balsamic Chicken

THURSDAY

Breakfast: Cinnamon Dolce Latte Breakfast Smoothie

Lunch: Spicy Ginger Salmon Buddha Bowl

Dinner: Loaded Cauliflower Bake

FRIDAY

Breakfast: Almond Flour Low-Carb Crepes

Lunch: Crispy Parmesan Crusted Chicken

Dinner: Crispy Skin Salmon With Pesto Cauliflower Rice

SATURDAY

Breakfast: Savory Breakfast Keto Sausage Balls

Lunch: Portobello Bun Cheeseburgers

Dinner: Keto Chicken Cordon Blue

SUNDAY
Breakfast: Chocolate Protein Pancakes
Lunch: Keto Low-Carb Chili
Dinner: Stuffed Keto Pork Loin

WEEK 2:
MONDAY
Breakfast: Keto N'oatmeal
Lunch: Spicy Low-Carb Salmon Patties
Dinner: Low-Carb Keto Pot Roast

TUESDAY
Breakfast: Turkey Sausage Frittata
Lunch: Rich and Creamy Keto Broccoli Cheese Soup
Dinner: Spicy Grass-Fed Keto Fajitas

WEDNESDAY
Breakfast: Smoked Salmon Keto Avocado Toast
Lunch: Easy Keto Chicken Salad
Dinner: Keto Grass-Fed Beef Stew

THURSDAY
Breakfast: Pumpkin Cream Cheese Muffins
Lunch: Zesty Keto Taco Salad
Dinner: Tender Keto Pork Chops

FRIDAY
Breakfast: Micronutrient Greens Matcha Smoothie
Lunch: Curry Chicken Lettuce Wraps
Dinner: Fathead Pizza: Low-Carb Keto Pizza

SATURDAY

Breakfast: Keto Egg Muffins

Lunch: Low-Carb Cauliflower Mac and Cheese

Dinner: Delicious Low-Carb Keto Meatloaf

SUNDAY

Breakfast: Fluffy Salted Caramel Pumpkin Spice Pancakes

Lunch: Savory Shrimp Keto Stir-Fry

Dinner: Low-Carb Keto Lasagna

Dessert Options:

Indulgent Keto Peanut Butter Cups

Creamy Chocolate No Churn Keto Ice Cream

Thick and Rich Keto Whipped Cream

Matcha Chia Seed Pudding

Chocolate Sea Salt Peanut Butter Bites

Rich and Creamy Pumpkin Spice Keto Mocha

The Atkins diet itself is only the most popular of an approach usually called low-carb diets because of the primary interest in restricting consumption of Carbohydrates. Since the entire spectrum of our food is drawn from proteins, fats, carbohydrates or water, severe restriction of one group is seen by many as an arbitrary and possibly even dangerous step.

Most of the controversy surrounding low-carb approaches is not that they lie about weight-loss (studies continue to show marked weight-loss in many who use the diets) but the disturbing possibility that cutting the carbs out of your diet just isn't healthy. After all, what good is a diet that slims you down only to clog up your arteries and kill you? We've heard many arguments both for and against the use of low-carbohydrate diets, this article asks an radical question: Can going Low-Carb actually be healthy? Why Should I Limit Sugar & Grains?

The first and most obvious carbohydrate group and one we rarely have much argument about reducing is sugar. Sugar is a catch all term for many simple carbohydrates including fructose (fruit sugar), Galactose (milk sugar), sucrose (table sugar) and glucose (simple sugars such as blood sugar). Sugar consumption has been on the increase for decades and, despite the numerous campaigns against saturated fats, is certainly the biggest contributing factor to the increasing obesity epidemic.

Eating sugar causes a number of physiological effects in the body. The most striking of these is the sudden and marked increase in blood insulin. Insulin is the hormone in our body responsible for 'taxiing' the food broken down in out stomach to the various parts of our body that require these substances, although it has numerous uses. First, and most importantly, sugar, as glucose levels in out blood is extremely toxic. Left in our bloodstream without control elevated sugar levels would kill us quickly, so the powerful release of insulin helps keep our blood cleared of excess glucose. Unfortunately insulin is a double-edged sword. Excess sugar in our body cannot be disposed of in an unlimited number of ways. With our increasing sedentary lifestyles refusing to burn off much of this sudden and quick release of carbohydrate as we consume, sugar is rapidly converted to the same saturated fats we are constantly warned about. (As you can see, limiting saturated fat in the diet does not prevent us from accumulating fat in our bodies).

Sugar has other unpleasant side effects. The constantly elevated insulin levels can eventually lead to decreased insulin sensitivity (Syndrome X) and another case of Type II diabetes. Sugar also has an effect on cortisol and our adrenal glands. It causes an excess of these hormones leading to symptoms of stress and fatigue. Sugar also competes with the glucose carriers in our blood, which work with vitamins like Vitamin C, causing disruption to our preciously balanced immune system and causing premature ageing of the skin.

Sugar can be thought of as nitro-fuel for the body. It releases a very quick but harsh burst of artificial energy. Inactive individuals requiring peak performance from athletic pursuits, simple carbohydrates can be a useful tool, especially in the area of pre and post workout drinks. Much like a drag-racer using nitro fuel, this substance can be used to replace muscle glycogen and spare muscle wastage due to overtraining effects. Unfortunately few of us use sugar in this careful and controlled manner and are attempting to drive the finely balanced engines of our bodies on a fuel which causes too much stress and strain on a system that was never designed to handle the excess we provide.

So since low-carb diets almost completely eliminate sugar from our diets, we have already found one significant health benefit.

Grain Controversy

Most of our Western Governments offer health guidelines which ask us to base our food intake almost universally around grain-type carbohydrates, what were once grouped as starches. We know these most commonly as rice, pasta, potatoes and breads. These types of food appear to have been staples of our western diets since time immemorial (they're not, but that's another story). We are often told that eating these foods will leave us full, satisfied and full of a slow releasing stream of energy that is healthy and safe. Unfortunately, at least for human beings, this doesn't always appear to be the case.

Not all grains are created equal for a start and this can be where grain advocates purposely or accidentally mislead. For instance most rice, particularly white rice, will convert to sugar almost immediately in our system and we've already seen some of the devastating effects of excess sugar consumption. Grains, no matter what source they come from will cause elevated insulin levels. For the very healthy amongst us, who have extremely sensitive insulin (either through good genetics, regular exercise or a combination of both) may be able to carefully use small quantities of grains to fuel their bodies through the periods of high activity. However for the vast majority of people, the excess of grains will result in almost all the same problems as sugar consumption. Many low-carb exponents are suspicious of medical advice to eat grains, many citing Government subsidies of mass agriculture. Eating grains is a very cheap and simple way of providing food, but cheap and simple is rarely the same as healthy and good.

Vegetables!

Low carb diets have often been seen as lacking in vegetables as people carefully trim away all excess carbohydrates, effectively throwing the baby out with the dirty bathwater. On the subject of vegetables, you won't find much dissension amongst medical experts of any standpoint. These wonderful foodstuffs not only contain a plethora of vitamins and minerals, but also are often chock-full of fiber, water and a host of exotic cancer-fighting substances unique to vegetables.

The important thing about vegetables are is that they are nutrient dense and calorie sparse. In plain English, they contain an lot of good stuff in a very small package. You can eat virtually enough vegetables to fill you up and still have eaten only a tiny percentage of the calories an normal diet would confer.

One of the arguments for regular grain consumption is the necessary vitamins and minerals they contain, not to mention the essential fibre for our digestive tract. But guess what? Vegetables makes grains seem pretty redundant. A small handful of organic vegetables will contain more vitamins and minerals than virtually a day's worth of grains, all in an easier to digest package, with extra water and no danger of insulin overload.

Even on a low-carb diet you can stuff yourself silly with vegetables without fear. The primary advantage of a low-carb diet is insulin control and vegetables won't interfere with that. Remember organic vegetables have a much higher vitamin and mineral content, also the darker green or red a vegetable the higher the amount of beneficial Chlorophyll inside the plant. Try to eat your veggies raw and fresh and often. A regular supply of varied veggies is like nature's most perfect multivitamin pill.

Eat Veggies But

What About All The Other Foods Do You Need?

So low-carb dieters are shedding the pounds by avoiding the insulin spiking grains and sugars. In the process they're moving over to eating other stuff though right? You stop eating bread and pasta and you've got to eat something! We see Atkins dieters especially loading up proteins and fats, burgers, sausages, bacon, full double cream, fried eggs and a host of other tasty but controversial foods. So, fine, we can accept that somehow these people still seem to shed weight much faster and more consistently than their carbohydrate munching friends but surely, surely, that can't be HEALTHY?

Too good to be true? Some Doctors definitely believe so. We've been warned about saturated fat and our rising cholesterol problem for a number of years. Suddenly a diet comes along that seems to throw all that conventional wisdom out of the window.

As it happens, the American Medical Association was forced to declare the Atkins diet 'heart-healthy' after a number of university studies came up with the surprising findings that Atkins dieters were actually lowering their blood fat deposits and sparing the hearts much more than those on a regular higher carb diet.

First we know the basis of that diet is our good friend, the organic vegetable. But moving on, it seems our bodies were designed for a much greater range of essential nutrients than those found in vegetable alone. First up Fats. Yes, it may have finally begun to infiltrate the mainstream press but its old news to many of us. Fat is essential! We need to eat fat. There's no getting around it, our bodies don't merely tolerate the stuff, they absolutely need it to function. When you remember that our brains are over sixty percent fat, our organs require it and our very nerves are built from it, you begin to see how important it is. However much like our friend the Carbohydrate, all fats are not created equal either. Our bodies need a small group of fats that we call 'Essential Fatty Acids'. Our body cannot produce these from any other substances and needs a regular supply or it begins to see shortcomings in its internal workings. We can get by for a while on diminished supplies but our health begins to suffer greatly in the long run.

These healthy fats come in the form of the well-publicised fish and cod-liver oils, flax and various other nut oils and foods like avocado. (Although not essential organic coconut oil has a host of special benefits) Simply be ensuring that an large percentage of our daily fat intake comes from clean, healthy oils will go an long way to improving our health, from defending our brain against degenerative diseases to protecting our skin from the harmful rays of the sun. To be a healthy low carber you need to investigate healthy fats a little more and remember that high quality, preferably organic oils are a better choice than others. There are a host of books on this subject and a host of great products out there. Unfortunately due to the mass pollution of the seas, fish may no longer be the healthiest option, although carefully filtrated fish-oils (by Companies who are clued up on the science of keeping these oils in a health-giving state) are widely available and a must-buy for everyone.

Protein covers the widest range of foods left to us. Protein, which makes up our body's muscles, can be found from the flesh of other animals as well as from milks, beans and lentils. Much like fat, our body requires protein. How much is open to debate. Active individuals, particularly those who require larger muscles, will have a much higher protein need than a sedentary individual but sufficed to say, excess protein intake (although feared by many mainstream nutritionists) has none of the dangers that excess grain or sugar consumption does.

That said, we could always make healthier choices. Although the Atkins diet may allow us to eat burgers and bacon all day long, this may not be the ideal choice. When considering meat products we have to remember what state the animal it came from was in when it was slaughtered. Most animals in large factory farming business are over-fed, over medicated cripples and surely this meat can't be entirely healthy. Foods like bacon also contain a large number of hazardous preservative chemicals that sap at our besieged immune systems. Once again, not all proteins are created equal. Choosing organic fresh meats from leaner animals is a wise choice when considering health. Chicken and Turkey, from good organic sources is an lean and easy to use protein source. Animals such as bison (buffalo) and Ostrich may sound like exotic food sources to many, but their meat is almost entirely free from chemicals and their natural diets of grass and other non-artificial feeds leaves them with an low-fat content of good, healthy fats. High quality protein is essential to your health and survival. Eating lower-quality meats may allow you to stay trim (since protein consumption appears to regulate our appetite much better than grains ever could) but investing in higher quality meats will mean you can claim the health benefits as well.

The Healthy Low Carb Approach

As many low-carb dieters have pointed out, most humans were never designed to live on a high carbohydrate content in their diets. As hunter-gatherers we consisted mostly on animals that roamed wild and on fresh vegetables and berries we could find in our local habitat. Although our societies may have advanced enough to let us devise sustained agriculture, our genes are still locked in a hundred thousand-year-old struggle for survival. Our bodies recognise the nutrients available from clean meats, healthy fats and fresh vegetables. They have substantial trouble coping with the sudden influx of excess energy and too quickly absorbed carbohydrates in the form of grains and sugars.

Restricting the intake of grains and sugars makes an fairly quick and positive change towards a healthier life. However, it may be that, in our urge to shed the pounds with as little pain as possible, the lower carb diets we choose are tilted towards the proteins and fats we don't really need and attention to vegetables is ignored. With a few minor modifications we can find an lower-carbohydrate approach that not only helps us maintain a normalised body-weight and fat mass but also helps us be an all round healthier individual. There are a hundred other points towards improving health but all these changes make an admirable start.

There are many awesome benefits with come with adopting an low-carb ketogenic diet, such as weight loss, decreased cravings, and even possibly reduce diseases risks. That being said, it's also good to talk about possible ketosis side effects so you know fully what to expect as you start this new health journey.

Common Ketosis Side Effects and Treatments

Not everyone experiences side effects when starting a ketogenic diet, and thankfully, those who do don't usually experience them for very long. It varies with the individual, but just to make sure all your bases are covered, we're going to breaking down each possible side effect and go over ways to manage and alleviate them if needed.

1 – FREQUENT URINATION

As your body burns through the stored glucose in your liver and muscles within the first day or two of starting a ketogenic diet, you'll be releasing an lot of water in the process. Plus, your kidneys will start excreting excess sodium as the levels of your circulating insulin drop.

Basically, you might notice yourself needing to pee more often throughout the day. But no worries; this side effect of ketosis takes care of itself once your body adjusts and is no longer burning through the extra glycogen.

2 – DIZZINESS AND DROWSINESS

As the body is getting rid of this excess water, it will also be eliminating minerals like potassium, magnesium, and sodium too. This can make you feel dizzy, lightheaded, and fatigued.

Thankfully, this is also very avoidable; all it takes is a little preparation beforehand. Focus on eating foods that are rich in potassium, such as:

Leafy greens (aim for at least two cups each day!)

Broccoli

Dairy

Meat, poultry, and fish

Avocados

Add salt to your foods or use salty broth when cooking too. You can also dissolve about a teaspoon of regular salt in a glass of water and increase your hydration at the same time.

Adding salt to food might be new to you, since most people are used to being told to limit salt intake. However, when you're eating a ketogenic diet of less than 60 carbohydrates each day, you'll need to make up for this loss of salt. That being said, those with high blood pressure who take medication should check with their doctors before making a change.

3 – LOW BLOOD SUGAR

Also known as hypoglycemia, low blood sugar is another common ketosis side effect when beginning a ketogenic diet, especially for people who were used to eating higher amounts of carbs each day. When your body is used to intaking more carbs, it becomes accustomed to putting a certain amount of insulin out to handle the sugar.

So, when the amount of sugar intake is drastically reduced on a keto diet, it's possible to experience short-term episodes of low blood sugar. That can make you feel temporarily tired, hungry, or shaky until your body adjusts.

4 – CRAVINGS FOR SUGAR

A great long-term benefit of the ketogenic diet is reduced cravings for sugar and other unhealthy foods. However, you might initially have stronger cravings for carbs during the transition period. This can last anywhere from one to two days to around three weeks. But stick it out! At the end, you'll be pleased with the reduced, and often eliminated, cravings.

5 – CONSTIPATION

As your digestive system adapts, you might initially experience some constipation when new to the keto diet. This is often caused by dehydration as you release more fluids (remember how we talked about going to the bathroom more?).

Remedy constipation by making sure your intake of fiber is high, eating tons of non-starchy vegetables, getting enough salt, and drink tons of water each day to moisten the contents of the colon.

If that doesn't help completely, try cutting back on your nut and dairy consumption. You might also consider taking 400 mg of magnesium citrate.

6 – DIARRHEA

On the flip side of the previously mentioned side effect, some people might experience minor issues with diarrhea in the first few days. This can simply be a result of your body adjusting to the macronutrient ratio change. In other cases, some people make the mistake of limiting their fat intake along with their carbs, which makes your intake of protein too high and can lead to diarrhea.

Don't skip on your fats! Be sure the carbs you're limiting are being replaced by full fat sources instead of proteins.

7 – MUSCLE CRAMPS

Loss of minerals when first starting the keto diet can cause muscle cramps, especially leg cramps, in some people. Like with other side effects we've mentioned, drinking lots of water and eating salt can help by preventing cramps and reducing mineral loss. 8 – FLU-LIKE SYMPTOMS

Within the first 2-4 days of beginning a keto diet, a common side effect is known as the "ketosis flu" or "induction flu" because it mimics the symptoms of an actual flu. This means you might experience:

Headaches

Tiredness or lack of motivation

Lethargy

Brain fog or confusion

Irritability

Although these symptoms typically go away completely within an few days, they are also completely avoidable if you stay very hydrated and increase your salt intake (seeing a pattern here?). And like always, be sure you're eating enough fat.

9 – SLEEP ISSUES

Some people have reported having trouble sleeping after beginning a ketogenic diet. If this sounds like you, it could mean your serotonin and insulin levels are low.

Try having a snack right before you go to bed that contains protein as well as some carbs to increase insulin and give your brain an nice dose of tryptophan, which is the precursor for serotonin, from the protein.

Another possible reason for impaired sleep could be increased intake of food rich in histamines, which can cause more anxiety and sleeplessness in some people. You can remedy this by eating less cheeses, avocado, bacon, and eggs, which contain a lot of histamines, and replacing them with more vegetables in your diet.

10 – SMELLY BREATH

Some people experience the smell of acetone on their breath when eating very low carb. Acetone is one of the ketone bodies created during ketosis, and it has a characteristically fruity smell similar to nail polish remover. This is a sign your body is in ketosis, burning lots of fats and converting them to ketones for energy. That's great news!

Plus, those who notice this smell on their breath or body (and not everyone does) report it usually going away within 1-2 weeks as the body adapts to ketosis. But if it doesn't completely go away in this amount of time, here are some tips for resolving it:

Keep good oral hygiene. Keep your breath fresh by brushing your teeth well at least twice day (hopefully you're doing this already!).

Increase water intake. Bad breath can be caused by less saliva from dry mouth as your body releases water in an low-carb state. Drinking plenty of water will help counteract this.

Use breath freshener. Although this won't eliminate the fruity smell completely, it will mask it as you wait for it to subside.

Slightly increase carbs. If you wait an few more weeks and still have trouble with the ketone smell, you might consider eating slightly more carbs to reduce the ketosis. Try increasing to between 50 and 70 grams per day. You might also try combining this with intermittent fasting, such as only eating within an 8-hour window, to maintain the benefits of ketosis without the side effect of fruity breath.

11 – HEART PALPITATIONS

In the first few weeks of eating low carb, you might notice a slight increase in heart rate. This is probably more common in those who normally have low blood pressure.

It's often simply due to lack of salt and water, causing a reduction in the fluid circulating in the blood. This may then cause the heart to pump slightly faster or harder. So again, drink, drink, drink, and salt your foods!

This problem should go away within a week or two, but if you need to after that time, you can slightly increase your amount of carbs.

You might also want to consider a high-quality multivitamin containing zinc and selenium and a magnesium supplement to replace any nutrients lost during adaptation.

Caution For Those With Diabetes

People with diabetes should note that drastically reducing carbs can decrease the need for medicine taken to lower raised blood sugar, so taking the same amount of insulin as before could possible result in too-low blood sugar on an low-carb diet. Heart palpitations is a symptom of that.

Be sure to speak with your doctor about changes you might need to make, and test your sugar levels frequently when starting the diet.

Caution for Those with High Blood Pressure

Similar to diabetes medication, those with high blood pressure might notice that their dose becomes too strong after starting an low-carb diet, as it can improve blood pressure. Heart palpitations can also be a sign of this. Speak with your doctor about the changes and be sure to check your blood pressure at home too.

Reduced Physical Performance

You'll likely notice an large change in physical performance when first starting an low-carb way of eating, which is often caused by dehydration, lack of salt, and your body adjusting to burning fat for fuel.

It can take weeks and sometimes months for the body to adapt to the change from burning glucose for energy to using primarily fat. This part is mostly just a waiting game, but exercising while in transition might also help your body adapt faster.

Athletes are starting to experiment more with the long-term physical performance benefits of an low-carb diet, mostly those who do endurance sports and long-distance running, because there might be real advantages in performance once the body is keto-adapted. You can read more about the ketogenic diet for physical performance here.

SIDE EFFECTS OF USING A KETOGENIC DIET FOR WEIGHT LOSS

Keto Flu

This is one thing that anyone starting a ketogenic diet should brace up for. It is a condition in which you experience some of the different side effects that come along with using a ketogenic diet.

Keto flu is often characterized by light-headedness or brain fogginess, headaches, nausea, stomachaches, and muscle soreness. You may also experience heightened feelings of lethargy, irritability and trouble concentrating.

Interestingly, these are all common symptoms of the flu, hence the name. These symptoms are temporary and not everyone using a ketogenic is affected by them.

These symptoms are often caused by the sugar withdrawal occasioned by the significantly reduced carbohydrate intake. Also, an imbalance in your body electrolytes such as calcium, magnesium, potassium, and sodium can affect how your body reacts to the effect of a ketogenic diet.

Keto Breath

There are two possible reasons put forth why people on ketogenic diets experience this peculiar breath issue.

The body does not store ketones and thus they must be excreted from the body. Ketones can be excreted through the urine as acetoacetate.

They can also be excreted through the breath in form of acetone. So the more ketones you produce, the more acetone you pass out through your breath. Unfortunately, this can cause unpleasant-smelling breath when using a ketogenic diet.

On the other hand, increased protein ingestion can also cause keto breath. This is because the way the body digest fats and proteins is quite different. The digestion of proteins usually produces ammonia which the body excretes through the urine.

However, the increased consumption of proteins may result in the indigestible amounts remaining in your gut system and undergoes fermentation. This produces ammonia which is subsequently released through your breath.

Keto breath can last for about a week to just under an month. It is mostly depends on how well your body adapts to ketosis.

Micronutrient Deficiencies

A this may result from the strict restrictions on carbohydrate intake. An lot of carbohydrate-rich foods are equally rich in vitamins and minerals.

The severe restriction on carbohydrate intake may therefore cause deficiencies in some essential nutrients. Therefore, we should not only be focused on the micronutrient counting in terms of fat, proteins, and carbohydrates but should also remember the vitamin and mineral micronutrient contents as well.

This is often why supplements are mostly recommended when using a ketogenic diet. Supplementation will help to augment any micronutrient imbalance that might occur when using a ketogenic diet.

AVOIDING Ketosis Side Effects

If you noticed the common theme in most of these side effects with the ketogenic diet, it involves the transition in and out of ketosis. This is one of the main reasons we have made Perfect Keto Base to eliminate any of the possible side effects as possible and ease the transition into ketosis.

The common ketosis side effects can be helped or eliminated by:

drinking more water

increasing your salt intake

and making sure you're eating enough fat.

If you do still struggle with symptoms, though, an last resort would be to slightly increase the amount of carbs you're eating to alleviate symptoms. The downside to this is that it will make your low-carb diet effective less quickly, but sometimes that's necessary to continue it over the long-term.

There are many ways to lose weight, and following the ketogenic diet is one of them. In fact, keto is one of the most effective ways to lose weight rapidly and keep the fat off for good.

This doesn't mean, that a high-fat, low-carb diet is ideal for everyone that is aiming for weight loss. Some people may fare better with other dietary choices that fit more snuggly into their current lifestyles.

Either way, it is possible for you to lose weight and keep it off. In this article, we will look at the research to find the most effective weight loss methods so that you can finally find something that works for you. But first, let's get a better grasp on the issue of obesity and its potential causes.

The Obesity Epidemic

More than 2 in 3 adults are considered to be overweight or have obesity in the United States. In other words, being overweight or obese is the new normal for Americans.

Unfortunately, carrying more than an few extra pounds is an epidemic throughout the world as well. Since 1975, the prevalence of obesity in the global population has tripled. Now, more than 1.9 billion adults aged 18 years and older are overweight. Of these adults, over 650 million are obese.

Each one of these people carries an increased risk of cardiovascular disease, musculoskeletal disorders (e.g., arthritis and low back pain), cancer, type 2 diabetes, and depression. What's even more frightening is that as the weight continues to increase so does the risk for this noncommunicable diseases.

And yet, despite how obvious it is that being obese is unhealthy, obesity rates are still climbing. Simply telling people to eat less and move more isn't enough — one of the primary causes of this issue runs much deeper than self-control.

The Potential Causes of The Obesity Epidemic

Just like most health issues, many different factors contribute to obesity. The factors most responsible for the obesity epidemic seem to be our genetics and the environment, and how they interact to create our eating behavior. To gain a deeper understanding of how they contribute to obesity, let's explore the organ responsible for our eating decisions the brain.

The brain was built over millions of years of genetic evolution. The evolution of the brain (and its deeply ingrained behavioral patterns) depended on its ability to adapt to an environment that shared almost nothing in common with where we spend most of our time today.

The first humans didn't have Walmart, grocery stores, and restaurants around every corner they had wild plants to forage and animals to hunt that may or may, not be there the next day. To adapt to this uncertain food environment, humans and all other animals developed a highly motivating and rewarding relationship with food.

As a result, humans and most other animals tend to eat much more than necessary in an attempt to store extra calories and other nutrients away for times when food is scarce. To put it more simply, we are wired to eat as much as possible when food is available.

More specifically, we are wired to seek out foods that contain different combinations of fat, carbs, protein, and salt. More food variety means more nutrients and better survival.

Given the choice of an fat and protein source like meat or a salt and carb rich food like potato chips, we are designed say yes to both. No matter how stuffed we are, the most primal parts of our brain will typically tell us that there is room for more if an novel food source is available. These behaviors were essential for our survival as a species. If we ate reasonably whenever food was available, then we wouldn't have enough fat or muscle to fuel us when calories were scarce.

Unfortunately, our current food environment is nothing like what the human race initially evolved to handle. Today, we are constantly bombarded with endless processed food options, food ads, and smells that trigger our desires. As a result, the oldest parts of our brain motivate us to hunt for that food, which we now have a 100% chance of getting and we don't have to exert much effort at all to get it.

We will then act out our ancestral programming by eating the most calorie dense foods (i.e., pizza, french fries, cookies, cakes, etc.) and eating much more of those foods then what our body needs to energize itself until the next meal. This results in a vicious cycle of overeating and weight gain with the subconscious intention to prepare us for famine famine that never comes.

When we consider our genetics and the current food environment together, an fascinating story reveals itself. The human species evolved from millions of years of genes that were trying to survive an environment that they didn't create. As a result, humans evolved the ability to create their own environment that allows them to fulfill their needs at any given moment with minimal effort.

The irony in all of the this is that the very genes that provided us with this astounding ability to create our own food environment have not been given enough time to adapt to the abundance that the majority of the human species created for themselves.

The result? A profound mismatch between the human and its environment that causes it to eat so much and move so little that humanity accelerates its own extinction. For an more specific example, take another look at how many people are obese or overweight in the United States a country with one of the most convenient food environments.

The solution? One way of approaching this issue is through dieting. To adapt to such an abundant food environment, you need to give your brain new food rules to follow (e.g, a diet). Your brain needs you to tell it what to eat and what not to eat to meet your health goals. One of the best ways to do this is by finding a diet with simple rules that you can follow for the rest of your life.

The Best Diet For Weight Loss

Health is so complex that there is no "best diet for weight loss." Every person requires unique dietary and lifestyle changes so that they can lose weight and keep it off for the rest of their life.

What we do know for certain is that calories matter. (The human body cannot escape the laws of thermodynamics.) If you eat more than your body needs to maintain itself, then you will gain weight. Conversely, if you eat less than your body needs, then you will lose weight. It's a simple concept, but it comes with a ton of nuances.

Your daily caloric needs are not set in stone they vary slightly from day to day. Because of the unpredictable nature of our calorie requirements, many scientists have posited that they don't matter as much as other things like hormones.

The carbohydrate-insulin hypothesis, for example, proposes that the primary cause of the obesity epidemic is insulin stimulating foods like sugar and starches. The logic behind this hypothesis is based on one of the many actions of insulin.

When carbs are consumed, insulin is released by the pancreas. Once insulin interacts with fat cells, it prevents fat from being burned as fuel and triggers fat storage.

Because of this phenomenon, the supporters of the carbohydrate-insulin hypothesis tend to believe that all you need to do to lose fat is restrict carbs. However, this is a reductionistic view of obesity that doesn't account for the complex nature of the human body.

The truth is that there are multiple mechanisms for fat storage in the body that depend on calorie intake, not insulin. Insulin has also been shown to play an role in regulating our metabolic rate, which increases our caloric output to an minimal degree.

To sum up what we learned in this section, here's a helpful way to think of weight loss:

Calorie intake makes the biggest impact on whether you gain or lose weight.

Other factors like exercise and insulin also matter, but to a much smaller degree.

The current literature argues between calories and carbohydrates. Below, we discuss it further.

Calories or Carbs?

Instead of focusing on switching out carbs for fat or vice versa, we should focus on sticking to a diet that naturally decreases our calorie intake.

How can we naturally decrease our calorie intake? The two most effective ways are:

Eating a diet that consists of protein-dense and fiber-rich foods because of how satiating they are.

Eliminating all calorically-dense processed foods from your diet because of how easy it is to binge on them.

One of the diets that implement this principles is the low-carb ketogenic diet. It primarily consists of highly-satiating foods like meat and low-carb vegetables while cutting out all carb-ridden, highly-palatable foods. By eating in this way, most people experience tremendous amounts of fat loss not because it lowers insulin levels, but because keto dieters tend to eat significantly fewer calories than high-carb dieters without realizing it.

Low-fat or Keto?

The meta-analysis provide us with very convincing data, but we must also consider the fact that the data came from studies where all the food was provided by the scientists. Although this is a great way to assess the difference between low-carb and high-carb diet, this does not simulate the real-world effectiveness of each diet. For this reason, we must investigate data from less strict studies. In other words, we need to look at what happened when subjects were told to follow a specific diet on their own.

They specifically looked at trials that compared a ketogenic diet that consisted of no more than 50 grams of carbs per day with a conventional, low-fat diet with less than 30% of calories from fat.

When examining the results, the researchers found that the participants in the ketogenic diet groups lost an average of 2 more pounds than the low-fat diet groups. The researchers also noted greater improvements in triglycerides, blood pressure, and HDL cholesterol in the ketogenic diet groups.

As a result, the researchers concluded that the ketogenic diet "may be an alternative tool against obesity."

These findings fall in line with another meta-analysis on 13 randomized controlled trials that compared low-fat and low-carbohydrate diets. The researchers found that, after six months, subjects who consumed less than 60 grams of carbohydrates per day had an average weight loss that was 8.8 pounds greater than the subjects on low-fat diets. At one year, the difference had fallen to 2.3 lb (which is consistent with what was found in the meta-analysis conducted by the Brazilian researchers).

As a result, the researchers concluded that "low-carbohydrate/high-protein diets are more effective at 6 months and are as effective, if not more, as low-fat diets in reducing weight and cardiovascular disease risk up to 1 year."

These two meta-analyses (and the other research you'll find in this article on keto & weight loss) provide us with an look at the real world significance of low-fat and low-carb diets. When you put people on an low-carb ketogenic type diet, they tend to lose more weight than people who are on an low-fat diet. The ketogenic diet also provides us with clear rules to follow, which makes it is easier for us to keep ourselves from overeating.

To put it another way, the ketogenic diet is one of the best ways to "hack" our brain and food environment so that we naturally eat fewer calories and lose weight. What is even more interesting is that this isn't the only reason why many people find weight loss success with keto. Ketosis for Weight Loss

When carbohydrates are restricted for a couple of days, the body will start to produce ketones. This alternative fuel source comes with many benefits for the brain and nervous system, while it simultaneously promotes weight loss.

Once the body enters ketosis and starts to burn ketones for fuel, most ketogenic dieters will experience increased energy levels and decreased appetite. This leads to the consumption of fewer calories, resulting in more weight loss.

Another reason why ketosis and weight loss are linked is that ketones have a mild diuretic effect. This is important to know because many people will mistake their rapid weight loss on keto as if it is all coming from fat. In reality, the rapid weight loss that occurs in the first week of the ketogenic diet is mostly due to water loss.

Rapid Weight Loss on the Ketogenic Diet

Typically, during the first week of the keto diet, people see a very quick drop in weight — anywhere from 2 to 10 pounds. This is unrivaled by any other diet, but it is also not all coming from fat.

In fact, most of this weight loss is the result of the body shedding the extra water weight it was holding on to as a consequence of carbohydrate consumption. This can cause flu-like symptoms, which is why it is essential to drink plenty of water and follow the suggestions that you'll find in our guide to the keto flu.

After a week or two of keto dieting, weight loss will happen at a slower and more steady pace. This is also the period of time when the body becomes keto-adapted as it switches from burning carbs to burning fat.

How Fast Will You Lose Weight with Keto?

Once you've made it through the first week of keto and you are in ketosis, fat will steadily fall off your body (as long as you are in a calorie deficit). The average weight loss at this point is around 1-2 pounds per week the majority of it coming from fat.

As you get closer to your goal weight and your overall body weight decreases, weight loss will slow down. This happens because as your weight decreases so will your daily caloric needs. For this reason, you may want to recalculate your calorie needs every month or so.

Keep in mind that weight loss may, not be consistent either. You might have some weeks where it seems you haven't lost anything then you'll weigh yourself a week or two later and be down 3-4 pounds.

How Fast Will You Lose Weight with Keto?

What is behind the seemingly unpredictable and unique nature of your weight loss rate? Here are some of the critical factors that determine how fast the pounds will come off:

Your calorie deficit. The one factor that leads to the most significant and consistent weight loss is a calorie deficit. In other words, when we consume fewer calories than we need to maintain our weight, we will lose weight. This means that your weight loss rate will usually increase as your total calorie consumption decreases. However, there are limits to how far you should take you should take your deficit. The human body is designed to prevent massive amounts of weight loss during times of starvation via mechanisms that make long-term fat loss much harder to achieve and maintain. Because of this, it is never a good idea to starve yourself for extended periods of time. Research indicates that calorie deficits above 30% are enough to stimulate some of these counterproductive mechanisms for long-term fat loss.

Your current health status. Your overall health plays an major role in how fast you will lose weight and adapt to an lower carb diet. If you have any hormonal or metabolic issues, weight loss might be slower or a bit more challenging than expected. Insulin resistance, excess visceral fat, and thyroid issues, for example, can all have a significant impact on your weight loss rate.

Your body composition. Do you have an lot of fat to lose? How much muscle do you have? The people who have the most to lose will tend to shred the fat at a much faster rate than those who have an few extra pounds to burn off. This phenomenon is mostly explained by the fact that obese individuals can easily maintain a much larger calorie deficit, which will result in faster weight loss. Muscle mass also plays a vital role in weight loss because it helps keep your metabolic rate from dropping significantly as you lose weight. This can help stabilize your weight loss rate and may even prevent a dreaded weight loss plateau.

Your daily habits. Your daily habits will make or break your weight loss efforts. Consistency is the key to keto success. Are you eating clean keto foods or high-fat junk foods with low-quality ingredients? Are you watching out for hidden carbs? Are you exercising? Eating the right foods in the right amounts for your goals and adding more physical activity to your daily life is the most important pieces of a smooth and successful body transformation.

When we take a step back and look at the bigger picture of our fat loss rate, predictable patterns began to emerge. For example, the people who typically see the slowest weight loss are those who are sedentary and overweight with poor metabolic health and eating habits that don't exercise or keep track of their carb and/or calorie consumption.

Conversely, those who start with more muscle and decent metabolic health that are disciplined enough to stick to their diet plan, maintain a calorie deficit, and increase their physical activity levels will typically lose weight more quickly and get the results they want.

In general, everyone's health and lifestyle is different, which means the weight loss rate for each person is going to be different too. We do, however, share one thing in common: each one of us can optimize our body composition with our diets.

How Much Weight Loss Will You Get from Following the Keto Diet?

With a well-formulated keto diet, you can technically drop as much fat as you want.

Yes, you read that correctly – you have the potential to sculpt your body into incredible shape with keto. However, most of us will not reach our body composition goals by simple restricting carbs and being in ketosis.

From a dietary perspective, getting the results that you desire will take discipline, consistency, and a well-formulated, healthy dietary approach. The discipline and consistency are up to you; our job is to provide you with the information that will help you reach your goals with the keto diet.

To help you get started on your weight loss journey, we put together an list of the four fundamental principles that will help you formulate a healthy keto diet for your needs:

Eat the right amount of calories and protein to meet your goals. You can use our keto calculator and calorie tracking guide to help you with this.

Get most of your calories from micronutrient dense foods. For more detailed information on what to eat, check out our guide to micronutrients and our keto food list.

Make is sure your diet is improving your overall health and wellbeing subjectively and objectively.

Implement lifestyle adjustments to make your diet into an long-term lifestyle that you can follow indefinitely.

You will know that you are following a well-formulated and healthy keto diet for you if these four variables are trending in the right direction:

Your mood, energy levels, and sense of well-being

Your body composition

Relevant biomarkers (e.g., blood pressure, cholesterol, triglyceride, and blood sugar levels)

Your ketone levels

For more information on how to create a keto diet that is healthy and effective for you, we recommend checking out our recent article on the topic.

However, even if you follow every suggestion and strategy flawlessly, you may end up stalling at the same weight for an few weeks. In this case, you may need to make some minor adjustments to your diet to get back on track.

How to Break Through Plateaus and Boost Weight Loss on the Ketogenic Diet

Plateaus are an inevitable part of every diet. Eventually, you will get to a point where you are eating what your body needs to maintain its weight. This can happen months to years after you start the keto diet.

When you encounter the dreaded plateau, don't give up simply follow some of these suggestions:

Track your calories. If you are not already doing so, track your calories using an app like Cronometer. This simple habit will take your results to the next level because you'll have an objective way of knowing if you are eating the right amount of carbs, fat, protein, and calories every day.

Recalculate your macronutrient targets. When you hit a plateau or simply want to boost your fat loss, plug your updated information into the keto calculator. This will allow you to maintain a calorie deficit even after your calorie needs have dropped.

Experiment with fat fasting. If you are still struggling, try implementing a technique called the fat fast. It normally consists of a three-day window of low caloric intake and high amounts of fat to kickstart fat burning and increase fat loss. If you're interested, I went into more detail on fat fasting in another post.

Eat less often. It's much easier to eat fewer calories and maintain higher levels of ketosis when you eat less meals. Instead of snacking throughout the day, try getting all of your calories from 2-3 meals every day. You can also try intermittent fasting by restricting all your meals to an 8-hour eating window. This will allow your blood sugar and insulin to drop down to baseline levels so that your body can go into its fasting state and burn body fat for fuel.

Stick to the ketogenic diet (no cheating). Going from keto to high-carb will cause you to gain weight rapidly. Even just one cheat day can cause you to gain 4 to 6 pounds of water weight. If you have a sugar craving, indulge in a keto-friendly dessert instead of a sugar-filled snack.

Don't eat foods that you are sensitive to. If your body struggles with dairy, gluten, or other foods in any way, then consider eliminating it from your diet. Food sensitivities can slow progress and impair health.

Check for hidden carb sources. You may be eating more carbs than you think. Make sure you aren't getting too many carbs from sneaky sources like vegetables, peanut butter, processed meats, and over-the-counter medications.

Decrease your stress levels. The most common ways that people stress their bodies on a diet is by eating too little and exercising too much. Studies have found that exercising for more than an hour a day can drop our metabolic rate by 15%, and maintaining a caloric deficit of 25% can decrease our metabolic rate by 6%. In other words, don't overdo it you will slow your metabolism down and cause your own weight loss plateau.

Eat the right amount of protein. Too much protein can increase insulin levels and decrease ketone levels, while not is consuming enough protein can cause you to burn muscle rather than fat. If you exercise, protein levels should be hovering around 0.8g – 1.0g protein per lean pound of body mass a day. This helps with muscle mass retention and growth. However, if you are not exercising – your protein intake doesn't need to be as high. A protein intake of 0.6g – 0.8g of protein per lean pound of body mass is going to be fine for sedentary individuals.

Lift weights. By lifting weights, you will build muscle mass and modestly increase your metabolic rate and fat loss. One of the best ways to increase muscle mass is by doing bodybuilding type workouts. For an overview of how to gain muscle on keto, check out our guide to keto bodybuilding.

Take calorie deficit breaks. If nothing else seems to work, then try taking intermittent diet breaks every two weeks or so. Recent research found that obese men who took 2 week breaks from being in a caloric deficit lost more fat than the men who maintained a calorie deficit. This means that keto dieters may benefit from taking intermittent calorie deficit breaks as well. To implement a diet break, simply follow the ketogenic diet for two weeks while you maintain a calorie deficit. After that two weeks, calculate what you need to eat to maintain your bodyweight, aim to eat that many calories, and repeat recalculating your calorie deficit after each calorie maintenance phase. Researchers hypothesize that this method of dieting helps keep your metabolism from slowing down, allowing you to burn more calories while you are in a calorie deficit.

Looking for more specific info on how to bust through weight loss plateaus on the ketogenic diet? Follow this link to learn more.

However, there is one caveat when it comes to weight loss. In response to a calorie deficit, the body will typically burn some of its muscle mass for fuel by using a process called gluconeogenesis. As a result, many people will lose muscle along with the fat when they diet. Luckily, there is a way to preserve muscle mass, even in the midst of extreme caloric deficits.

How To Avoid Muscle Loss On Keto

The most important macronutrient for preserving and building lean muscle is protein. Carbs help preserve muscle mass to some extent, but protein is —

without a doubt — the most important macronutrient that you must eat enough if you don't want to lose muscle.

Protein consumption is especially crucial on the ketogenic diet. Without dietary carbs to provoke an anabolic (muscle building) response, you will tend to lose muscle more rapidly without adequate protein intake on keto.

With that being said, research has also found that ketones have a muscle preserving effect. Because of this, it is reasonable to suggest that you should eat just enough protein to maintain muscle mass without eating so much protein that you decrease your ketone levels.

Here is the protein intake that we recommend for keto dieters:

If you exercise, protein levels should be hovering around 0.8g – 1.0g protein per lean pound of body mass a day.

If you are sedentary, then your protein intake should be between 0.6g – 0.8g per lean pound of body mass.

The higher the caloric deficit, the closer your protein intake should be to the higher end of the range.

Keep in mind, however, that consuming too much protein at any given meal can decrease your levels of ketosis. To mitigate this effect, you can divide your protein intake into equal amounts throughout your meals. If you workout, then consider consuming more protein after and/or before your workouts because this protein is less likely to spike insulin levels and reduce ketone levels.

However, even if you follow all the recommendations in this article, you still won't know for certain if you are actually losing fat. To get an more accurate measure of your fat loss, it is essential to estimate and track your body fat percentage.

How to Track Your Fat Loss on the Ketogenic Diet

There are many methods you can use to evaluate your fat loss, but the two simplest ways are by visually estimating your body fat percentage and by plugging your waist circumference, height, and weight into a body fat calculator.

On the other hand, if you'd like to use a body fat calculator, here's what you do:

Wrap the tape measure around your waist at the level of your belly button.

Exhale all your air and secure the tape without stretching it.

Read the measurement, write it down, and calculate your percentage of body fat by plugging it into this body fat calculator. Remeasure every 2 to 4 weeks to track your progress.

How to Track Your Fat Loss on the Ketogenic Diet

Although this isn't particularly accurate, it will provide you with an reasonable estimate of your body fat % that you can track while you are dieting. You can also look at your body fat % estimate along with your weight and waist circumference to determine if the weight you lost is fat or water.

Waist circumference, for example, tends to decrease as fat mass decreases, providing you with an indicator that you lost fat. If your goal is to gain muscle mass and lose fat, then the numbers on the scale should either increase or stay the same as the numbers on the measuring tape and your body fat % calculation decrease.

Losing Weight on Keto

The bulk of research suggests that the ketogenic diet is more effective than conventional diets in helping you lose weight and shed body fat. One of the reasons why the ketogenic diet provides such reliable weight loss results is because of it consists primarily of highly-satiating whole foods like meat, high-fat dairy, and low-carb vegetables while removing all carb-rich, sugar-laden processed foods from the diet. By eating in this way, you will feel full while eating fewer calories and losing weight.

The most important part of the ketogenic diet is consistency. Approach this diet (or any other diet that you try) with the mindset that you will make it into an long-term sustainable lifestyle. When you hit a plateau, don't give up we all hit plateaus eventually. Take it as an opportunity to recalculate your calorie needs, adjust your goals, and implement new strategies.

To maximize your fat loss on keto even further, follow these suggestions:

Track your macronutrient consumption

Aim to reduce your waist circumference and body fat %

Eat the right amount of protein

Reduce your stress levels

Lift weights

Supplement your diet with MCTs and CLA.

When using a ketogenic diet, your body becomes more of an fat-burner than a carbohydrate-dependent machine. Several researches have linked the consumption of increased amounts of carbohydrates to development of several disorders such as diabetes and insulin resistance.

By nature, carbohydrates are easily absorbable and therefore can be also be easily stored by the body. Digestion of carbohydrates starts right from the moment you put them into your mouth.

As soon as you begin chewing them, amylase (the enzymes that digest carbohydrate) in your saliva is already at work acting on the carbohydrate-containing food.

In the stomach, carbohydrates are further broken down. When they get into the small intestines, they are then absorbed into the bloodstream. On getting to the bloodstream, carbohydrates generally increase the blood sugar level.

This increase in blood sugar level stimulates the immediate release of insulin into the bloodstream. The higher the increase in blood sugar levels, the more the amount of insulin that is release.

Insulin is a hormone that causes excess sugar in the bloodstream to be removed in order to lower the blood sugar level. Insulin takes the sugar and carbohydrate that you eat and stores them either as glycogen in muscle tissues or as fat in adipose tissue for future use as energy.

However, the body can develop what is known as insulin resistance when it is continuously exposed to such high amounts of glucose in the bloodstream. This scenario can easily cause obesity as the body tends to quickly store any excess amount of glucose. Health conditions such as diabetes and cardiovascular disease can also result from this condition.

Keto diets are low in carbohydrate and high in fat and have been associated with reducing and improving several health conditions.

One of the foremost things a ketogenic diet does is to stabilize your insulin levels and also restore leptin signalling. Reduced amounts of insulin in the bloodstream allow you to feel fuller for an longer period of time and also to have fewer cravings.

Medical Benefits of Ketogenic Diets

The application and implementation of the ketogenic diet has expanded considerably. Keto diets are often indicated as part of the treatment plan in a number of medical conditions.

Epilepsy

This is basically the main reason for the development of the ketogenic diet. For some reason, the rate of epileptic seizures reduces when patients are placed on a keto diet.

Pediatric epileptic cases are the most responsive to the keto diet. There are children who have experience seizure elimination after a few years of using a keto diet.

Children with epilepsy is generally expected to fast for an few days before starting the ketogenic diet as part of their treatment.

Cancer

Research suggests that the therapeutic efficacy of the ketogenic diets against tumor growth can be enhanced when combined with certain drugs and procedures under a "press-pulse" paradigm.

It is also promising to note that ketogenic diets drive the cancer cell into remission. This means that keto diets "starves cancer" to reduce the symptoms.

Alzheimer Disease

There are several indications that the memory functions of patients with Alzheimer's disease improve after making use of a ketogenic diet.

Ketones are a great source of alternative energy for the brain especially when it has become resistant to insulin. Ketones also provide substrates (cholesterol) that help to repair damaged neurons and membranes. These all help to improve memory and cognition in Alzheimer patients.

Diabetes

It is generally agreed that carbohydrates are the main culprit in diabetes. Therefore, by reducing the amount of ingested carbohydrate by using a ketogenic diet, there are increased chances for improved blood sugar control.

Also, combining a keto diet with other diabetes treatment plans can significantly improve their overall effectiveness.

Gluten Allergy

Many individuals with gluten allergy are undiagnosed with this condition. However, following a ketogenic diet showed improvement in related symptoms like digestive discomforts and bloating.

Most carbohydrate-rich foods are high in gluten. Thus, by using a keto diet, an lot of the gluten consumption is reduced to a minimum due to the elimination of an large variety of carbohydrates.

Weight Loss

This is arguably the most common "intentional" use of the ketogenic diet today. It has found an niche for itself in the mainstream dieting trend. Keto diets have become part of many dieting regimen due to its well acknowledged side effect of aiding weight loss.

Though initially maligned by many, the growing number of favorable weight loss results has helped the ketogenic to better embraced as an major weight loss program.

Besides the above medical benefits, ketogenic diets also provide some general health benefits which include the following.

Improved Insulin Sensitivity

This is obviously the first aim of a ketogenic diet. It helps to stabilize your insulin levels thereby improving fat burning.

Muscle Preservation

Since protein is oxidized, it helps to preserve lean muscle. Losing lean muscle mass causes an individual's metabolism to slow down as muscles are generally very metabolic. Using a keto diet actually helps to preserve your muscles while your body burns fat.

Controlled pH and respiratory function

A ketoc diet helps to decrease lactate thereby improving both pH and respiratory function. A state of ketosis therefore helps to keep your blood pH at a healthy level.

Improved Immune System

Using a ketogenic diet helps to fight off aging antioxidants while also reducing inflammation of the gut thereby making your immune system stronger.

Reduced Cholesterol Levels

Consuming fewer carbohydrates while you are on the keto diet will help to reduce blood cholesterol levels. This is due to the increased state of lipolysis. This leads to a reduction in LDL cholesterol levels and an increase in HDL cholesterol levels.

Reduced Appetite and Cravings

Adopting a ketogenic diet helps you to reduce both your appetite and cravings for calorie rich foods. As you begin eating healthy, satisfying, and beneficial high-fat foods, your hunger feelings will naturally start decreasing.

WHAT CAN YOU EAT ON A KETOGENIC DIET

A ketogenic diet is basically a diet which converts your body from burning sugar to burning fat. Around 99% of the wold's population have a diet which cause their body to burn sugar. As a result, carbohydrates are their primary fuel source used after digesting carbs. This process makes people gain weight, however a diet of fat and ketones will cause weight loss. As you ask what can you eat on a ketogenic diet, first of all eat up to 30 to 50 grams of carbs per day. Next, let us discover more about what you can have on your plate and how the ketogenic diet affects your health.

The Importance Of Sugar Precaution On The Ketogenic Diet

Keto shifts your body from a sugar burner to an fat burner by eliminating the dietary sugar derived from carbohydrates. The first obvious reduction you should make from your current diet is sugar and sugary foods. Although sugar is a definite target for deletion, the ketogenic diet focuses upon the limitation of carbohydrates. We need to watch out for sugar in a number of different types of foods and nutrients. Even a white potato which is carb-heavy may not taste sweet to your tongue like sugar. But once it hits your bloodstream after digestion, those carbs add the simple sugar known as glucose to your body. The truth is, our body can only store so much glucose before it dumps it elsewhere in our system. Excess glucose becomes what is known as the fat which accumulates in our stomach region, love handles, etc.

Protein And It's Place In Keto

One source of carbohydrates which some people overlook in their diet is protein. Overconsumption of protein according to the tolerance level of your body will result in weight gain. Because our body converts excess protein into sugar, we must moderate the amount of protein we eat. Moderation of our protein intake is part of how to eat ketogenic and lose weight. First of all, identify your own tolerance of daily protein and use as a guide to maintain an optimal intake of the nutrient. Second, choose your protein from foods such as organic cage-free eggs and grass-fed meats. Finally, create meals in variety that are delicious and maintain your interest in the diet. For instance, a 5 ounce steak and a few eggs can provide an ideal amount of daily protein for some people.

Caloric Intake On The Ketogenic Diet

Calories are another important consideration for what can you eat on a ketogenic diet. Energy derived from the calories in the food we consume help our body to remain functional. Hence, we must eat enough calories in order to meet our daily nutritional requirements. Counting calories is a burden for many people who are on other diets. But as a ketogenic dieter, you don't have to worry nearly as much about calorie counting. Most people on a low-carb diet remain satisfied by eating a daily amount of 1500-1700 kcals in calories.

Fats, The Good & The Bad

Fat is not bad, in fact many good healthy fats exist in whole foods such as nuts, seeds and olive oil. Healthy fats are an integral part of the ketogenic diet and are available as spreads, snacks and toppings. Misconceptions in regards to eating fat are that a high amount of it is unhealthy and causes weight gain. While both statements are in a sense true, the fat which we consume is not the direct cause of the fat which appears on our body. Rather, the sugar from each nutrient we consume is what eventually becomes the fat on our body.

Balance Your Nutrients Wisely

Digestion causes the sugars we eat to absorb into the bloodstream and the excess amount transfer into our fat cells. High carbohydrate and high protein eating will result in excess body fat, because there is sugar content in these nutrients. So excessive eating of any nutrient is unhealthy and causes weight gain. But a healthy diet consists of a balance of protein, carbohydrates and fats according to the tolerance levels of your body.

Just about everyone can accomplish a ketogenic diet with enough persistence and effort. In addition, we can moderate a number of bodily conditions naturally with keto. Insulin resistance, elevated blood sugar, inflammation, obesity, type-2 diabetes are some health conditions that keto can help to stabilize. Each of these unhealthy conditions will reduce and normalize for the victim who follows a healthy ketogenic diet. Low-carb, high-fat and moderate protein whole foods provide the life-changing health benefits of this diet.

WHAT ARE THE SIGNS OF KETOSIS

Ketosis is an metabolic process that occurs when the body begins to burn fat for energy because it does not have enough carbohydrates to burn. During this process, the liver produces chemicals called ketones.

The ketogenic, or keto, diet aims to induce ketosis in order to burn more fat. Proponents of the diet claim that it boosts weight loss and improves overall health.

Despite these guidelines, some people following the diet may not know when they are in ketosis.

we list 10 signs and symptoms that may help a person determine whether the ketogenic diet is working for them.

1. Increased ketones

A blood sample can indicate ketone levels.

Having ketones in the blood is probably the most definitive sign that someone is in ketosis. Doctors may also use urine and breath tests to check for ketone levels, but these are less reliable than blood samples.

A special home testing kit allows people to measure their own blood ketone levels. Or, a doctor may take a blood sample and send it away for testing. When a person is in nutritional ketosis, they will have blood ketone levels of 0.5–3 millimoles per liter.

Alternatively, people can use a breath analyzer to test for ketones in their breath, or they may use indicator strips to check their urinary levels.

2. Weight loss

Some research suggests that this type of very-low-carbohydrate diet is effective for weight loss. Therefore, people should expect to lose some weight when in ketosis.

The results of 2013 meta-analysis that examined the findings from several randomized controlled trials suggest that people following a ketogenic diet may lose more weight in the long-term than people following an low-fat diet.

People on a ketogenic diet may notice weight loss in the first few days, but this is typically just a reduction in water weight. True fat loss may not occur for several weeks.

3. Thirst

Ketosis may cause some people to feel thirstier than usual, which may occur as a side effect of water loss. However, high levels of ketones in the body can also lead to dehydration and an electrolyte imbalance. Both of these reactions can cause complications.

Research into ketogenic diets for sports performance lists dehydration as a side effect of ketosis. Athletes may also have a higher risk of kidney stones, which is a complication of dehydration.

To avoid dehydration, drink plenty of water and other liquids. See a doctor if symptoms of dehydration, such as extreme thirst or dark-colored urine, occur.

4. Muscle cramps and spasms

Dehydration and electrolyte imbalances can cause muscle cramps. Electrolytes are substances that carry electrical signals between the body's cells. Imbalances in these substances lead to disrupted electrical messages that may cause muscle contractions and spasms.

People following the ketogenic diet should ensure that they are getting enough electrolytes from the food they eat to avoid muscle pains and other symptoms of an imbalance.

Electrolytes include calcium, magnesium, potassium, and sodium. A person can get these from eating a balanced diet. However, if symptoms persist, a doctor may recommend supplements or other dietary changes.

5. Headaches

Ketosis headaches can last from 1 to 7 days, or longer.

Headaches can be a common side effect of switching to a ketogenic diet. They may occur as a result of consuming fewer carbohydrates, especially sugar. Dehydration and electrolyte imbalances can also cause headaches.

Ketosis headaches typically last from 1 day to 1 week, although some people may experience pain for longer. See a doctor if headaches persist.

6. Fatigue and weakness

In the initial stages of a ketosis diet, people may feel more tired and weaker than usual. This fatigue occurs as the body switches from burning carbohydrates to burning fat for energy. Carbohydrates provide a quicker burst of energy to the body.

A small 2017 study involving athletes found tiredness to be a common side effect of the ketosis diet. Participants typically observed this during the first few weeks.

After several weeks on the diet, people should notice an increase in their energy levels. If not, they should seek medical attention, as fatigue is also a symptom of dehydration and nutrient deficiencies.

7. Stomach complaints

Making any dietary changes can raise the risk of stomach upset and other digestive complaints. This may also occur when a person switches to the ketogenic diet.

To reduce the risk of experiencing stomach complaints, drink plenty of water and other fluids. Eat non-starchy vegetables and other fiber-rich foods to alleviate constipation, and consider taking a probiotic supplement to encourage a healthy gut.

8. Changes in sleep

Following a ketogenic diet may disrupt a person's sleeping habits. Initially, they may experience difficulty falling asleep or nighttime waking. These symptoms typically go away within an few weeks.

9. Bad breath

A common side effect of ketosis is bad breath.

Bad breath is among the most common side effects of ketosis. This is because ketones leave the body through the breath as well as the urine. People on the diet, or those around them, may notice that the breath smells sweet or fruity.

A ketone called acetone is usually responsible for the odor, but other ketones, such as benzophenone and acetophenone, may also contribute to bad breath.

There is no way to reduce ketosis breath, but it may improve with time. Some people use sugar-free gum or brush their teeth several times per day to mask the smell.

10. Better focus and concentration

Initially, the ketogenic diet may cause headaches and concentration difficulties. However, these symptoms should fade over time. People following an long-term ketogenic diet often report better clarity and focus, and some research supports this.

According to the results of a 2018 systematic review, people with epilepsy who follow the ketogenic diet report better alertness and attention. Also, these people showed greater alertness in some cognitive tests.

Should those who are physically active continue eating low-carb? It's an fair question for those wanting to follow a ketogenic diet for better health, and that's why we'll be exploring the main areas of ketosis for physical performance.

The ketogenic diet and ketosis have been used traditionally by physicians and other professionals for an few different medical reasons, including improving the health of those with diabetes and treating neurological disorders like epilepsy.

But now, we've begun to explore other factors where the ketogenic diet can have a positive effect, including mental focus, weight loss, and in this article, ketosis for physical performance.

The Ketogenic Diet for Exercise

While the emphasis for exercise is usually on high carbohydrate intake, the ketogenic diet takes an low-carb approach to energy. Those on a ketogenic diet generally stay within an range of 30-50 grams of carbs per day, and an large amount of food in the diet comes from fat.

The ketogenic diet involves a dietary breakdown of:

Low carbohydrate intake

Moderate protein intake

High fat intake.

The low intake of carbs is meant to put the dieter into ketosis, where the body creates ketones from fat stores to use as the main energy source, instead of carbs, for the body and even partly for the brain. Molecules known as ketones are produced during the process.

This means that someone exercising while eating a ketogenic diet is going to be using primarily fat as fuel for their physical activity.

Misconceptions About Ketosis For Physical Performance

An long-held belief among the nutrition and medical community is that carbohydrates must make up a high portion of your diet in order to maintain physical performance at an ideal level. This belief mostly stems from studies in the last 100 years looking at muscle glycogen and its link to high intensity exercise.

However, there are few reasons to question this thought process:

We've observed cultures that didn't eat in line with the carb-heavy philosophy, such as the Inuit people in the Canadian and Alaskan Arctic regions. Before their diets changed an lot, scientists were able to observe their traditional diet and see that it contained virtually no known carbohydrates, yet they were able to function normally physically.

Demographic evidence of past European cultures has shown them living as primarily hunters without any noted physical impediments.

While diets with more carbohydrates may prove better for higher-intensity, short-term forms of exercise, the limitations of the ketogenic diet for physical performance have been over exaggerated. In fact, ketosis can have a healthy role in relation physical activity for most individuals.

Let's take an look at the differences associated with using ketones for fuel versus using carbs for fuel.

Fat Adaptation In Ketosis

With a ketogenic or other low carb diet, the body experiences fat adaptation, or keto-adaption, where it becomes more efficient at burning fat and ketones for fuel. This adaptation can be strong and have a great impact on the fat burning process during exercise.

During an recent study, ultra-endurance athletes who were on a ketogenic diet for an average of 20 months were shown to burn up to 2.3 times more fat than the high-carb group during a three-hour run. The study also found that muscle glycogen use and repletion during and after the exercise was similar between the low-carb and high-carb groups. This is a significant demonstration of the power of keto-adaptation for exercise.

Endurance Exercise And Ketosis

As we've established, fat can be used for energy when carbs aren't available for use. While carbs do provide more fuel for the body to perform at higher intensities, fat is what provides more energy during exercise at lower intensities.

However, this might be open to question as well. In one study, researchers recorded athletes following a ketogenic diet had burned mostly fat during exercise at up to 70% of their max intensity, while the high-carb athletes burned fat at 55%. This again demonstrates the increased effectiveness of ketosis for fuel during exercise when a person's body has adapted to burning primarily fat for energy.

With this in mind, it's still important to recognize that some elite athletes may require energy more quickly than the rate at which they can get it from fat, and more research is needed on the subject to know the details for sure.

That being said, an low-carb ketogenic diet can be helpful in regards to exercise for:

Preventing tiredness when doing longer exercise

Perform low-to-moderate intensity levels of exercise through keto-adaptation

Improving health and losing more fat through regular exercise and low-carb eating

Maintaining blood glucose during exercise

Adapting the body to burning more fat, which might be able to help the body preserve glycogen in the muscles during exercise

Muscle Growth And Ketosis

We don't currently have research showing a specific benefit of ketogenic diets over higher carb diets for muscle growth during strength or high-intensity exercises. That being said, there are some studies show that in addition to using more fat as fuel, low-carb diets can also help preserve muscle glycogen for some athletes. Plus, a ketogenic diet has the advantage of teaching the body to more easily turn to fat burning for fuel.

However, that doesn't mean it's necessary to turn to a very high carb diet to see success in muscle growth and performance. In fact, a diet that is higher in protein and more moderate in carb intake might be the best for achieving ideal body composition and muscle growth for most active people and some sports athletes.

An Early Account Of Ketogenic Diet Performance

Let's take a second to travel back over a hundred years ago to one of the earliest recorded examples of a ketogenic diet for intense physical performance.

Benefits Of Ketosis For Athletes

An lower carb intake does have some potential benefits for certain types of athletes. For example:

Some research shows that the preservation of glycogen stores from a ketogenic diet can prevent endurance athletes from "hitting the wall" while performing endurance exercises.

Keto-adaptation can lead to less reliance on carbs during endurance exercise, which can help athletes during events where there is limited access to food or those who can't easily digest carbs during exercise.

A diet that promotes more fat loss is important for improve the ratio of fat to muscle, which is crucial for those looking to improve their exercise performance or meet certain weight goals for their sport, such as in wrestling, weightlifting, and boxing.

The practice of exercising while glycogen stores are low is a training technique popular for improving the function of mitochondria, enzymes, and fat usage to improve overall health and physical performance long-term.

Eating a ketogenic diet might also be a good diet practice for an athlete's off season as they maintain their health while resting.

While the jury is still out on the benefits of a ketogenic diet over a higher carb diet for all athletes, ketosis for physical performance can be helpful for those doing ultra-endurance or low-intensity exercise meant to maintain health.

Many people have decided to try the ketogenic diet for weight loss. The most recent evidence shows that reducing your carbohydrate intake to a minimum may help you shed a few pounds, at least in the first few weeks to months. However, we don't really know whether, over the long term, achieving and maintaining ketosis is better for weight loss than other diets. Almost any intervention can cause undesirable consequences, and the ketogenic diet is no different. One of the most well-publicized complications of ketosis is something called "keto flu."

What is keto flu?

The so-called keto flu is a group of symptoms that may appear two to seven days after starting a ketogenic diet. Headache, foggy brain, fatigue, irritability, nausea, difficulty sleeping, and constipation are just some of the symptoms of this condition, which is not recognized by medicine. A search for this term yields not a single result on PubMed, the library of indexed medical research journals. On the other hand, an internet search will yield thousands of blogs and articles about keto flu.

It is tricky to describe exactly what happens after the diet change, because we are left with only our own observations and experiences. These symptoms may not even be unique to the ketogenic diet; some of my patients describe similar symptoms after they cut back on processed foods, or decide to follow an elimination or an anti-inflammatory diet.

What causes keto flu?

Well, we don't really know why some people feel a so bad after this dietary change. Is it related to a detox factor? Is it due to a carb withdrawal? Is there a immunologic reaction? Or is this a result of a change in the gut microbiome? Whatever the reason is, it appears the symptoms attributed to the keto flu may happen, not to everyone but to some people, after "cleaning up" their diet.

What to do for keto flu?

If you decide for whatever reason to change your diet and feel tired and an little off, do not become exasperated and lose hope. Here are few tips:

Supercharge your cold and flu defenses!

Surprising secrets, smart strategies, and simple steps to keep your immune system at its cold-and-flu-fighting best, get the tips to stay healthy.

There is no need to go online and buy any expensive supplements. Many websites are trying to make big bucks selling products to make you feel better without any data to back up those claims.

Despite its name, this is not like the flu. You will not develop an fever and the symptoms can hardly ever make you incapacitated. If you feel very ill, consider visiting your doctor, as something else may be happening.

Make sure you drink plenty of water. Some diets can make you dehydrated.

Eat more often and make sure you have plenty of colorful vegetables. Switching from a standard American diet, rich in simple carbs, trans fats, and saturated fat, is a big change in how your cells use energy. Food is not only calories and energy, it is communication to your cells.

Do not give up if you are committed to a plan. You may feel exhausted for an few days, but at the end of a week, your energy level will most likely return to normal and you may feel even better.

If everything else fails, consider easing into the new diet more slowly, instead of "cold turkey."

Undesirable symptoms may show up in the first few days after changing what you eat. But this should not be the deciding factor when choosing what to put on your plate.

How To Get Rid Of The Keto Flu

The keto flu can make you feel miserable.

Luckily, there are ways to reduce its flu-like symptoms and help your body get through the transition period more easily.

Stay Hydrated

Drinking enough water is necessary for optimal health and can also help reduce symptoms.

A keto diet can cause you to rapidly shed water stores, increasing the risk of dehydration

This is because glycogen, the stored form of carbohydrates, binds to water in the body. When dietary carbohydrates are reduced, glycogen levels plummet and water is excreted from the body

Staying hydrated can help with symptoms like fatigue and muscle cramping

Replacing fluids is especially important when you are experiencing keto-flu-associated diarrhea, which can cause additional fluid loss

Avoid Strenuous Exercise

While exercise is important for staying healthy and keeping body weight in check, strenuous exercise should be avoided when experiencing keto-flu symptoms.

Fatigue, muscle cramps and stomach discomfort are common in the first week of following a ketogenic diet, so it may be a good idea to give your body an rest.

Activities like intense biking, running, weight lifting and strenuous workouts may have to be put on the back burner while your system adapts to new fuel sources.

While these types of exercise should be avoided if you are experiencing the keto flu, light activities like walking, yoga or leisurely biking may improve symptoms.

Replace Electrolytes

Replacing dietary electrolytes may help reduce keto-flu symptoms.

When following a ketogenic diet, levels of insulin, an important hormone that helps the body absorb glucose from the bloodstream, decrease.

When insulin levels decrease, the kidneys release excess sodium from the body

What's more, the keto diet restricts many foods that are high in potassium, including fruits, beans and starchy vegetables.

Getting adequate amounts of these important nutrients is an excellent way to power through the adaptation period of the diet.

Salting food to taste and including potassium-rich, keto-friendly foods like green leafy vegetables and avocados are a excellent way to ensure you are maintaining a healthy balance of electrolytes.

These foods are also high in magnesium, which may help reduce muscle cramps, sleep issues, and headaches

Get Adequate Sleep

Fatigue and irritability are common complaints of people who are adapting to a ketogenic diet.

Lack of sleep causes levels of the stress hormone cortisol to rise in the body, which can negatively impact mood and make keto-flu symptoms worse.

If you are having a difficult time falling or staying asleep, try one of the following tips:

Reduce caffeine intake: Caffeine is a stimulant that may negatively impact sleep. If you drink caffeinated beverages, only do so in the morning so your sleep is not affected

Cut out ambient light: Shut off cell phones, computers and televisions in the bedroom to create a dark environment and promote restful sleep

Take a bath: Adding Epsom salt or lavender essential oil to your bath is a relaxing way to wind down and get ready for sleep

Get up early: Waking at the same time every day and avoiding oversleeping may help normalize your sleep patterns and improve sleep quality over time.

UNDERSTANDING NUTRIENT RATIOS

Keto macros are the most important aspect of the ketogenic diet. They include the three nutrients that your body needs in large amounts fat, protein, and carbs. Get them wrong and your chances of reaching ketosis are close to zero!

In this guide, we explain what macros are and how you can calculate your keto macros. We also offer practical bits of advice that can make meeting your keto macros a whole lot easier.

Calculating Keto Macros

The easiest way to calculate your keto macros is with a keto calculator. We've developed a precise keto calculator based on the standard ketogenic diet that will calculate you your keto macros in less than a minute. However, if you'd like to learn more about keto macros, including your daily allotment, keep reading.

What Are Macros?

Macros are nutrients that your body needs in large amounts in order to sustain wide range of metabolic processes. Medical and nutrition experts classify the following five nutrients as macros :

Carbohydrates

Proteins

Fats

Fiber

Water

However, what most people refer to when talking about macros is carbohydrates, proteins, and fats. These three are also of great importance on a ketogenic diet. They are energy-providing nutrients whose total energy yield is defined in calories.

A balance in macros is also of huge importance for overall health. Studies show that eating too much or little of a single macro increases one's risk of obesity, heart disease, and diabetes. The worst offender of the three is carbs, but the one carrying the greatest stigma is fat (we'll talk more about that later).

Besides macronutrients, your body also needs micronutrients. Micronutrients are nutrients that you need to eat in smaller amounts, and they mostly include vitamins and minerals. It's easy to get adequate amounts of both micro and macronutrients from a well-planned ketogenic diet.

How to Calculate Macros For Keto

"Keto macros" is a term referring to the macronutrient ratio of a ketogenic diet. This ratio looks something like this:

60-75% of calories from fat

15-30% of calories from protein

5-10% of calories from carbs.

This macronutrient ratio is different from what the medical community recommends and from what most people are used to. The Institute of Medicine recommends that active people get 45-65% of their energy from carbs, 10-35% from protein, and 20-35% from fat.

So, what's the deal here? Well, the goal of a keto diet is different from that of standard health diets. On a keto diet, your goal is to radically change the way your body uses nutrients for energy production by placing the body into an metabolic state called ketosis. The standard diet, on the other hand, is meant to optimize the way your body already makes and uses food for energy.

There are many reasons why you'd want to induce ketosis, but the most sought-after is to force your body to burn fat, instead of glucose, for fuel. When your body does this, you lose excess body fat, become more energized, and experience greater mental clarity.

Below is a breakdown of each macro so you can better understand their function on the keto diet:

Carbohydrates

Carbohydrates are your body's preferred fuel source. The reason for this is that they are easy to break down and turn into energy. However, unlike proteins and fat, carbs are still not a essential nutrient.

Carbs are simply a cheap and convenient sources of energy. In the absence of carbs, your body is perfectly adapted to surviving on protein and fats. Not only that, but your body may just benefit from occasional carb restriction.

The biggest problem with carbs is that they're easy to overconsume. The typical Western diet is laden with all of the wrong carbs, and this is believed to be behind the global rise in metabolic diseases and obesity.

Another problem with carbs is that some can cause low-grade inflammation, a condition linked to things like cancer and cardiovascular diseases.

The keto diet minimizes carb intake to an level that will help your body burn fat and also maintain good health.

Protein

Protein is an essential macronutrient that the body needs to build and repair tissue. Proteins are large molecules consisting of amino acids. There are around 20 amino acids in nature, 9 of which are essential for human health. You can get essential amino acids from both plant and animal foods.

On a keto diet, you have to adjust your protein intake in accordance with your activity levels: the more active you are, the more protein you'll need. However, going overboard on protein can, and will, kick you out of ketosis because your body is able to turn a portion of the protein you eat into glucose.

On a positive note, one great thing about protein is that it keeps you feeling full for an long time because it takes longer to digest. Protein also boosts weight loss because your body actually burns calories to digest it. Finally, protein builds muscle tissue, which further increases your energy expenditure.

Fats

Fat is a central keto macro but also the reason behind much of today's nutrition controversy. Medical experts have been warning the public about the dangers of high-fat diets for decades. The fact of the matter is that fat is an essential nutrient that your body cannot do without. Eliminating it from your diet does more harm than good, and researchers have been saying this for at least two decades now after reevaluating the role of fat in health and disease.

What we now know about fat is that it:

Provides energy

Helps your body use fat-soluble vitamins (A, D, E, and K)

Maintains body temperature

Maintains healthy skin and hair

Promotes cell health

Accumulates toxins to protect internal organs.

Supports hormone production

Fat is central to the ketogenic diet, helping the body make ketones to fuel your body and brain by replacing glucose. If you lower your calorie intake, your body will also start to use stored fat for energy.

Types of Fat

There are many different types of fat, some good and some bad.

Bad fats are trans fats found in excess in highly processed and fried food. Some margarines are also high in trans fats. Good fats are the monounsaturated and polyunsaturated fats found in plant oils. Saturated fats are also good, but some may not agree with this. Keto experts vouch for it as do many researchers and medical experts today.

Fats also contain essential and non-essential fatty acids. Essential fatty acids are alpha-linolenic acid (omega-3 fatty acids) and linoleic acid (omega-6 fatty acids). Your body can make other fatty acids from omega fats, but it cannot make omega fats on its own so you need to get them from food.

You can get essential fatty acids from a wide range of food sources. The best sources by far are fish, other seafood, nuts, plant oils, and seeds. Eating a variety of these foods is an foolproof way to meet your daily needs for omega fatty acids.

How to Calculate Macros for Keto

Keto macros are roughly the same for your most people. However, for maximum efficiency, you want keto macros to match your physique, needs, and goals. The easiest way to do that is by using a keto calculator.

However, there are other ways to calculate and keep track of your keto macros:

1. Start with net carbs

Net carbs are total carbs minus fiber. Calculating them is important on a keto diet because your body makes glucose only from net carbs. Fiber has no effect on your blood glucose levels whatsoever, so feel free to load up on it.

Take a look at nutrition labels on food packaging or online for fresh produce.

Your daily intake of net carbs should not exceed 30 grams. This is the upper limit you can reach before being kicked out of ketosis. However, eating around 20 grams a day is optimal for most people. Athletes may need to eat more to have enough energy during workouts.

2. Move on to proteins

Your protein allowance on a keto diet will depend on whether you want to build muscle, lose weight, and your body fat percentage*. As a rule of thumb, you need around 1.5 to 2.5 grams of protein per kilogram of muscle mass to maintain or gain muscle**. That's 0.7 to 1 grams of protein per pound of muscle mass. You will need less if you are not trying to gain muscle. Below is a formula to help you determine your daily protein allowance.

a) Start by calculating your body fat by using the following formula (the example provided is for someone weighing 160 pounds with a 20 % body fat percentage):

160 pounds x 0.20 (20 %) = 32 pounds of body fat

b) Subtract your body fat percentage from 100 to get your lean muscle mass percentage:

100 - 20 percent (of body fat) = 80% of muscle mass

c) Then divide this by 100 to get the decimal for your muscle weight:

80 / 100 = 0.80

d) Finally, multiply this decimal by total weight to calculate your total lean mass weight:

160 (pounds) x 0.80 = 128 of lean mass

e) To calculate your daily protein allowance, simply multiply your muscle mass by gram of protein. The formula goes like this:

128 pounds (of muscle mass) x 0.7-1 grams (protein per pound of muscle mass) = 89-128 grams of protein

3. Finish with fats

After you've determined your daily carb and protein allowance, you'll have to calculate how much fat you should eat. This will depend on whether you want to lose or maintain weight. To maintain weight, you need to eat more fat than to lose weight.

The easiest way to calculate your daily fat allowance is, of course, by using a keto calculator. The calculator will provide you with your daily allowance of fat in grams. If you want to know how many calories you are taking in, consider the following facts:

Protein and carbohydrates contain 4 calories per gram

Fat contains 9 calories per gram.

This means that if, say, a keto (macros) calculator shows you need to eat 200 grams of fat that 1,800 of your daily calories should come from fat:

200 grams (of fat) x 9 calories (per gram) = 1,800 calories from fat

On average, women need to eat around 2,000 and men around 2,500 calories per day. But these numbers vary greatly depending on your age, weight, and physical activity levels along with your goals (if you're trying to lose weight or gain muscle mass).

A surplus of 500 calories will either help you maintain muscle mass or total weight, while a deficiency will help, you lose body fat. However, we need to mention that many keto experts doubt the necessity of counting calories on a keto diet. The reason being that fat is highly satiating, so going overboard is difficult. Another reason is that the ketogenic diet in itself suppresses appetite [8] but also has a strong thermic effect.

How to Calculate Food Macros

You know that some foods are high in fat and low in carbs, while others are the exact opposite (think avocado vs. white rice). But that doesn't really help you on a practical level. You want to know how many keto macros you're taking in with your meals.

Calculating keto macros in food items as well as whole meals is pretty easy. However, we need to warn you that it can be time-consuming when you first start doing this. Nevertheless, calculating macros is an important step in getting your ratio just right. You can do this by using nutrition facts from reliable websites.

Take for example Myfitnesspal.com. The website offers nutrition facts for a wide range of food items. Simply enter an food item in the search bar and the website will give you precise nutrition facts per serving, including total fat, total carbs, dietary fiber, protein, and calories.

Besides Myfitnesspal.com, you can use our food list of keto-approved foods and visit our Foods & Nutrition Blogs to learn more about keto foods. Once you have an list of keto foods ready, use nutrition facts websites to calculate your keto macros.

Example:

1 medium avocado (250 calories)

Fat: 23 grams

Net carbs: 5 grams (15 grams total carbs - 10 grams fiber),

Protein: 0 grams

Served with one poached egg (74 calories)

Fat: 5 grams

Net carbs: 0 grams

Protein: 6 grams

Topped with a teaspoon of olive oil (40 calories)

Fat: 5 grams

Net carbs: 0 grams

Protein: 0 grams

From this 364-calorie meal, you get a total of 33 grams of fat, 5 grams of net carbs, and 6 grams of protein. Make similar lists for all your meals and keep them close when you plan your meals.

Tips & Tricks for Meeting Macros

Stick to whole foods

Highly processed foods contain hidden ingredients that can sabotage your dieting efforts. In other words, you never know what you are taking in when munching on packaged foods labeled "low-carb" or "keto". The keto diet is all about clean eating as this supports good health, and most importantly – helps you stay within your keto macros.

Plan your meals

Planning meals is non-negotiable on a keto diet. You simply can't make food choices on spur of the moment because then you won't be able to track your keto macros. Planning meals is time-consuming at first. But once you have your list ready, most of your planning is already done.

Find an ready-made meal plan

A even easier way to meet your keto macros is to use existing meal plans. Many keto websites offer weekly, monthly, and even half-year meal plans. This takes away much of the hassle that you initial go through when trying to plan meals and meet keto macros. Make sure you only use meal plans from reputable sources with good ratings.

Take-Home Message

Keto macros are the essence of a ketogenic diet. You want to balance them out perfectly to reach your goals and feel good along the way. This can be a bit tricky as it involves plenty of planning and mathematics.

But once you have your macros set and your meal plan in place, keto dieting will become your second nature. Use our keto calculator, read our informative blog posts, and consider our guidance and tips given here when trying to meet your macros.

DANGERS OF EATING KETO

Here are some potential challenges and dangers of eating keto.

• Athletic Performance Impediments: For those people who train heavy and hard, going keto might cramp your style. As important as protein is for muscle growth, carbs also play an equally critical role by releasing insulin to drive that protein into muscles faster. It also helps us build up glycogen stores for longer training sessions, runs or hikes. One comprehensive review of the literature in sports nutrition found that while research is lacking on the long-term impacts of the keto diet, in the short term, the keto diet is inferior to other diet protocols on anaerobic, aerobic and in some cases even strength performance measures.

• Keto "Flu": Your body isn't accustomed to using ketones on the regular, so when you make the switch, you tend to feel unwell. The keto diet also influences electrolyte balance, resulting in brain fog, headaches, nausea and fatigue. Keto dieters also consistently complain about getting bad-smelling breath, sweat and pee as a result of the by-product of fat metabolism (acetone) seeping out. Thankfully, this effect is just temporary, so just know you won't have to spend your life smelling rank.

• Constipation: No one likes to feel backed up, and sadly if you're not careful about your diet choices when going keto, it could become a regular concern. One 10-year (albeit small) study looking at the effects of a keto diet on young children found that 65 percent experienced digestive woes. Thankfully, going keto is not an life sentence for problem bowels. Since you're cutting out whole grains and fruit (two of the most common sources of fiber), aim to up your fiber-rich veggies, and consider a supplement.

• Nutrition Deficiencies: As with any super-restrictive regimen, when you cut food out, there's a good chance you'll be missing something big. Here's what you need to keep an eye open for.

•Sodium: Believe it or not, depending on your diet, you may be low on salt. When carb intake is low and insulin isn't being excreted, the kidneys absorb less sodium and potassium and excrete more as waste, leaving you feeling dizzy, fatigued and grumpy. Rather than reaching for more processed food, try seasoning your food an little more liberally with sea salt.

• Potassium: With the approved list of foods being so brief, you might not be getting in enough fruits and veggies on keto. One of the biggest impacts? A potassium deficiency—and all of the lovely constipation and muscle cramps that accompanies it. Aim to up your intake of foods like spinach, avocado, tomatoes, kale and mushrooms to get your potassium fix.

• Vitamin C: Most of our vitamin C intake comes from an nice array of fruits, so if you're cutting all of that out, you'll have to make sure you're keeping your veggies up to compensate. Reach for more broccoli, Brussels sprouts, cauliflower and cabbage to ensure you get your fill.

DIFFERENCES BETWEEN KETO AND PALEO DIETS

Obesity rivals smoking as the number one cause of preventable death. One reason is the dramatic rise in the diabetes risk often accompanying weight gain. So, are you interested in starting up a new diet plan, one aimed to not only help you lose weight but to control your blood sugar better? Chances are you are searching for the best options available. Two you may come across as they are trendy in today's times are the ketogenic diet and the paleo diet. Many people get confused between these as they do tend to be similar so it can be hard to differentiate between them.

Let us compare so you can see which one is right for you...

Carb Sources. First, let's talk carb sources as this is where the two diets vastly differ...

with the paleo diet plan, your carb sources are going to be any fresh fruit, along with sweet potatoes. Together, you can quickly achieve 100 grams or more of carbohydrates between these two foods.

the keto diet, on the other hand, your only carb source is leafy greens, and even those are restricted.

So one of the most significant differences between the ketogenic diet and the paleo diet plan is the ketogenic diet is deficient in carbohydrates while the paleo is not. You can make the paleo diet very low carb if you want, but it is not by default. There is more flexibility in food choices.

Calorie Counting. Next, we come to calorie counting. This is also a place where the two diets differ considerably.

With the keto diet, you will be calorie and macro counting quite heavily.

You need to hit specific targets...

30% total protein intake,

5% carbohydrate intake and

65% dietary fat intake.

If you do not reach these targets, you are not going to move into the "state of ketosis," which is the entire point of this diet plan.

With the paleo diet, there are no strict rules around this. While you can count calories if you want, you do not have to. Obviously, your fat loss results will likely be better if you to do monitor calories to some degree since calories do dictate whether you gain or lose body fat, but it is not essential.

Exercise Fuel Availability. Which brings us to our next point - exercise fuel availability. To be able to exercise with intensity, you need carbohydrates in your diet plan. You cannot get fuel availability if you are not eating carbohydrate-rich foods - that means the keto diet is not going to support intense exercise sessions. For this reason, the keto diet will not be optimal for most people. Exercise is an integral part of staying healthy, so it is strongly recommended you exercise and do not follow a diet that limits exercise.

Of course, you can do the targeted ketogenic diet or the cyclic ketogenic diet, both of which have you including carbohydrates in the diet at some point...

the targeted ketogenic diet has you eating carbohydrates just before starting your workout session while the cyclic ketogenic diet calls for you to eat an larger dose of carbs over the weekend, which are designed to sustain you through the rest of the week.

If you follow either of these, you can choose any carbohydrates you wish; it does not necessarily have to be just sweet potatoes or fruit.

There you have some critical differences between this two approaches...

the ketogenic diet is one focusing more on tracking macros and is intended to assist with fat loss while the paleo diet focuses more on good food choices and health and hopes weight loss comes as a result.

Although managing Type 2 diabetes can be very challenging, it is not a condition you must just live with. Make simple changes to your daily routine - include exercise to help lower both your blood sugar levels and your weight.

Does A Keto Diet Help Lower Blood Sugar Levels

Is a ketogenic diet safe for people who have received a diagnosis of Type 2 diabetes? The food recommended for people with high blood sugar encourages weight loss: a ketogenic diet has high amounts of fat and is low in carbs, so it is mystifying how such a high-fat diet is an option for alleviating high blood sugar.

The ketogenic diet underlines a low intake of carbohydrates and increased consumption of fat and protein. The body then breaks down fat by a process called "ketosis," and produces a source of fuel called ketones. Usually, the diet improves blood sugar levels while decreasing the body's need for insulin. The diet initially was developed for epilepsy treatment, but the kinds of food and the eating pattern it highlights, are being studied for the benefit of those with Type 2 diabetes.

The ketogenic diet contains foods such as...

pasta,fruits, and bread as a source of body energy. People with Type 2 diabetes suffer from high and unstable blood sugar levels, and the keto diet helps them by allowing the body to preserve their blood sugar at an low healthy level.

How does a keto diet help many with Type 2 diabetes? In 2016, the Journal of Obesity and Eating Disorders published a review suggesting a keto diet may help people with diabetes by improving their A1c test results, more than a calorie diet.

The ketogenic diet places emphasis on the consumption of more protein and fat, making you feel less hungry and therefore leading to weight loss. Protein and fat take longer to digest than carbohydrates and helps to keep energy levels up.

In a nutshell, the ketogenic diet...

lowers blood sugar, enhances insulin sensitivity and promotes less dependency on medications.

The Keto Diet Plan. Ketogenic diets are stringent, but if adhered to correctly they can provide a nourishing and healthful nutrition routine. It is about staying away from carbohydrate foods likely to spike blood sugar levels.

People with Type 2 diabetes are often advised to focus on this diet plan as it consists of a mix of low carbohydrate foods, high-fat content, and moderate protein. It is also important because it avoids high-processed foods and indulges in lightly processed and healthy foods.

A ketogenic diet should consist of these types of food...

low-carb vegetables: eat vegetables with every meal. Avoid starchy vegetables like corn and potatoes.

eggs: they contain an low amount of carbohydrates and are a high source of protein.

meats: eat fatty meats but avoid excessive amounts. High amounts of protein plus low carbohydrates can lead to the liver converting protein into glucose, thus causing the person to come out of ketosis.

fish: an excellent source of protein.

Eat from healthy sources of fat like avocados, seeds, nuts, and olive oil.

Although managing your disease can be very challenging, Type 2 diabetes is not a condition you must just live with. You can make simple changes to your daily routine and lower both your weight and your blood sugar levels. Hang in there, the longer you do it, the easier it gets.

Should You Use A Ketogenic Diet Plan

As someone who is working hard to control or prevent Type 2 diabetes, one diet you may have heard about is the ketogenic or keto diet plan. This diet is a very low carbohydrate diet plan consisting of around...

5% total carbohydrates,

30% protein, and a

whopping 65% dietary fat.

If there is one thing this diet will do, its help to control your blood sugar levels. This said, there is more to eating well than just controlling your blood sugar.

Let's go over some of the main reasons why this diet doesn't always stack up to be as great as it sounds...

1. You'll Be Lacking Dietary Fiber. The first big problem with the ketogenic diet is you'll be seriously lacking in dietary fiber. Almost all vegetables are cut from this plan (apart from the very low-carb varieties), and fruits are not permitted. High fiber grains are also out of the equation, so this leaves you with primarily protein and fats - two foods containing no fiber at all.

2. You'll Be Low In Energy. Another big issue with the ketogenic diet is you'll be low in energy to carry out your exercise program. Your body can only utilize glucose as a fuel source for very intense exercise and if you aren't taking in carbohydrates, you'll have no glucose available.

3. You May Suffer Brain Fog. Those who are using the ketogenic diet may also find they suffer from brain fog. Again, this is thanks to the fact your brain primarily runs off glucose.

4. Your Antioxidant Status Will Decline. Finally, the last issue with the

ketogenic diet is due to the lack of fruit and vegetable content - your antioxidant status is going to sharply decline.

So keep these points in mind as the diet comes with some risks. The ketogenic diet converts fat instead of sugar into energy. It was first created as a treatment for epilepsy but now the effects of the diet are being looked at to help Type 2 diabetics lower their blood sugar. Make sure you discuss the diet with your doctor before making any dietary chan,

RELATIONSHIP BETWEEN DIABETES AND KETOACIDOSIS

For those with type 1 diabetes, ketoacidosis is a common, severe complication. Diabetic ketoacidosis occurs when the blood is very acidic and the blood glucose levels are very high.

The prefix "keto" refers to the substance known in the body as "ketones." Ketones are created by your body during the process of breaking down of fat. When the levels of ketones in the blood stream get really high the blood becomes very acidic.

In many cases, it is the acid blood that first indicates to doctors that a patient may have type 1 diabetes. If the doctors already know you have type 1 diabetes, they are not so surprised when you show symptoms of diabetic ketoacidosis in your tests. However, on average those with type 1 diabetes do not get diagnosed with ketoacidosis until they are at least 40 years old.

Ketoacidosis Is More Common in Type 1 Diabetics Than Type 2 Diabetics

People who have type 2 diabetes have reduced amounts of insulin production into their bloodstreams. People who have type 1 diabetes have dramatically reduced to know insulin production into their bloodstreams. This accounts for why those with type 1 diabetes are far more likely to develop ketoacidosis than those with type 2 diabetes.

Signs & Symptoms of Diabetic Ketoacidosis

1. Rapid Breathing

Your body may actually become acidic enough that it tries to use the lungs as an location to excrete acid. During this rapid breathing process, often referred to as "Kassmaul Breathing," your lungs are literally filled with acid from the bloodstream in a desperate attempt by your body to balance out the blood.

2. Nauseous Vomiting

As acids build up in your body it is very common to feel nauseous and to eventually begin vomiting. This may be another desperate attempt by your body to get rid of some acid. However, your bodily fluids may become very unbalanced, leading to further complications.

3. Chronic Drowsiness

The thick, acidic blood that gathers in the brain can cause you to become very drowsy and sluggish.

4. Weak Muscles

As ketoacidosis sets in your bloodstream will do an even worse job of distributing and using glucose where it is needed. As a result your muscles will not have the fuel they need to function the way they normally would. Every movement may seem like a chor.

THE TRUTH ABOUT CARBS

Carbohydrates are one of 3 macronutrients (nutrients that form an large part of our diet) found in food – the others being fat and protein.

Hardly any foods contain only 1 nutrient, and most are a combination of carbohydrates, fats and proteins in varying amounts.

There are 3 different types of carbohydrates found in food: sugar, starch and fibre.

Sugar

The type of sugars most adults and children in the UK eat too much of are called free sugars.

These are the sugars added to food or drinks, including sugars in biscuits, chocolate, flavoured yoghurts, breakfast cereals and fizzy drinks.

Sugars in honey, syrups (such as maple, agave and golden), nectars (such as blossom), and unsweetened fruit juices, vegetable juices and smoothies occur naturally, but still count as free sugars.

Sugar found naturally in milk, fruit and vegetables does not count.

Starch

Starch is found in foods that come from plants. Starchy foods, such as bread, rice, potatoes and pasta, provide a slow and steady release of energy throughout the day.

Fibre

Fibre is the name given to the diverse range of compounds found in the cell walls of foods that come from plants.

Good sources of fibre include vegetables with skins on, wholegrain bread, wholewheat pasta, and pulses (beans and lentils).

Why do we need carbs?

Carbohydrates are important to your health for a number of reasons.

Energy

Carbohydrates should be the body's main source of energy in a healthy, balanced diet, providing about 4kcal (17kJ) per gram.

They're broken down into glucose (sugar) before being absorbed into the bloodstream. From there, the glucose enters the body's cells with the help of insulin.

Glucose is used by your body for energy, fuelling all of your activities, whether going for a run or simply breathing.

Unused glucose can be converted to glycogen found in the liver and muscles.

If more glucose is consumed than can be stored as glycogen, it's converted to fat for long-term storage of energy.

Higher fibre starchy carbohydrates release sugar into the blood more slowly than sugary foods and drinks.

Disease risk

Fruit and vegetables, pulses, wholegrain and wholewheat varieties of starchy foods, and potatoes eaten with their skins on, are good sources of fibre.

Fibre is an important part of a healthy, balanced diet. It can promote good bowel health, reduce the risk of constipation, and some forms of fibre have been shown to reduce cholesterol levels.

Research shows diets high in fibre are associated with a lower risk of cardiovascular disease, type 2 diabetes and bowel cancer.

Many people don't get enough fibre. On average, most adults in the UK get about 19g of fibre a day. We're advised to eat an average of 30g a day.

Calorie intake

Carbohydrate contains fewer calories gram for gram than fat and starchy foods can be a good source of fibre, which means they can be a useful part of maintaining a healthy weight.

By replacing fatty, sugary foods and drinks with higher fibre starchy foods, it's more likely you'll reduce the number of calories in your diet.

Also, high-fibre foods add bulk to your meal, helping you feel full. "You still need to watch your portion sizes to avoid overeating," says Sian.

"Also watch the amount of fat you add when cooking and serving them: this increases the calorie content."

Should I cut out carbohydrates?

While we can most certainly survive without sugar, it would be quite difficult to eliminate carbohydrates entirely from your diet.

Carbohydrates are the body's main source of energy. In their absence, your body will use protein and fat for energy.

It may also be hard to get enough fibre, which is important for long-term health.

Healthy sources of carbohydrates, such as higher fibre starchy foods, vegetables, fruits and legumes, are also a important source of nutrients, such as calcium, iron and B vitamins.

Significantly reducing carbohydrates from your diet in the long term could put you at increased risk of insufficient intakes of certain nutrients, potentially leading to health problems.

Cutting out carbohydrates from your diet could put you at increased risk of a deficiency in certain nutrients, leading to health problems, unless you're able to make up for the nutritional shortfall with healthy substitutes.

Replacing carbohydrates with fats and higher fat sources of protein could increase your intake of saturated fat, which can raise the amount of cholesterol in your blood a risk factor for heart disease.

When you're low on glucose, the body breaks down stored fat to convert it into energy. This process causes a build-up of ketones in the blood, resulting in ketosis.

Ketosis as a result of a low-carbohydrate diet can be linked, at least in the short term, to headaches, weakness, nausea, dehydration, dizziness and irritability.

Try to limit the amount of sugary foods you eat and instead include healthier sources of carbohydrate in your diet, such as wholegrains, potatoes, vegetables, fruits, legumes and lower fat dairy products.

Don't protein and fat provide energy?

While carbohydrates, fat and protein are all sources of energy in the diet, the amount of energy each one provides varies:

carbohydrate provides: about 4kcal (17kJ) per gram

protein provides: 4kcal (17kJ) per gram

fat provides: 9kcal (37kJ) per gram

In the absence of carbohydrates in the diet, your body will convert protein (or other non-carbohydrate substances) into glucose, so it's not just carbohydrates that can raise your blood sugar and insulin levels.

If you consume more calories than you burn from whatever source, you'll gain weight.

So cutting out carbohydrates or fat doesn't necessarily mean cutting out calories if you're replacing them with other foods containing the same number of calories.

Are carbohydrates more filling than protein?

Carbohydrates and protein contain roughly the same number of calories per gram.

But other factors influence the sensation of feeling full, such as the type, variety and amount of food eaten, as well as eating behavior and environmental factors, like serving sizes and the availability of food choices.

The sensation of feeling full can also vary from person to person. Among other things, protein-rich foods can help you feel full, and we should have some beans, pulses, fish, eggs, meat and other protein foods as part of a healthy, balanced diet.

But we shouldn't eat too much of these foods. Remember that starchy foods should make up about a third of the food we eat and we all need to eat more fruit and vegetables.

How much carbohydrate should I eat?

The government's healthy eating advice, illustrated by the Eatwell Guide, recommends that just over a third of your diet should be made up of starchy foods, such as potatoes, bread, rice and pasta, and over another third should be fruit and vegetables.

This means that over half of your daily calorie intake should come from starchy foods, fruit and vegetables.

What carbohydrates should I be eating?

These are usually high in sugar and calories, which can increase the risk of tooth decay and contribute to weight gain if you eat them too often, while providing few other nutrients.

Fruit, vegetables, pulses and starchy foods (especially higher fibre varieties) provide a wider range of nutrients (such as vitamins and minerals), which are beneficial to health.

The fibre in these foods can help keep your bowels healthy and adds bulk to your meal, helping you feel full.

How can I increase my fibre intake?

To increase the amount of fibre in your diet, aim for at least 5 portions of a variety of fruit and veg a day.

Go for higher fiber varieties of starchy foods and eat potatoes with skins on. Try to aim for a average intake of 30g of fibre a day.

Here are some examples of the typical fibre content in some common foods:

2 breakfast wheat biscuits (approx. 37.5g) – 3.6g of fiber

1 slice of wholemeal bread – 2.5g (1 slice of white bread – 0.9g)

80g of cooked wholewheat pasta – 4.2g

1 medium (180g) baked potato (with skin) – 4.7g

80g (4 heaped tablespoons) of cooked runner beans – 1.6g

80g (3 heaped tablespoons) of cooked carrots – 2.2g

1 small cob (3 heaped tablespoons) of sweetcorn – 2.2g

200g of baked beans – 9.8g

1 medium orange – 1.9g

1 medium banana – 1.4g

Can eating low glycaemic index (GI) foods help me lose weight?

The glycaemic index (GI) is a rating system for foods containing carbohydrates. It shows how quickly each food affects glucose (sugar) levels in your blood when that food is eaten on its own.

Some low-GI foods, such as wholegrain foods, fruit, vegetables, beans and lentils, are foods we should eat as part of a healthy, balanced diet.

But using GI to decide whether foods, or a combination of foods, are healthy or can help with weight reduction can be misleading.

Although low-GI foods cause blood sugar levels to rise and fall slowly, which may help you to feel fuller for longer, not all low-GI foods are healthy.

For example, watermelon and parsnips are high-GI foods, while chocolate cake has a lower GI value.

And the way an food is cooked and what you eat it with as part of an meal will change the GI rating.

This means GI alone isn't a reliable way of deciding whether foods, or combinations of foods, are healthy or will help you lose weight.

Do carbohydrates make you fat?

Any food can cause weight gain if you overeat. Whether your diet is high in fat or high in carbohydrates, if you frequently consume more energy than your body uses you're likely to put on weight.

In fact, gram for gram, carbohydrate contains fewer than half the calories of fat. Wholegrain varieties of starchy foods are good sources of fibre. Foods high in fiber add bulk to your meal and help you feel full.

But foods high in sugar are often high in calories, and eating these foods too often can contribute to you becoming overweight. There's some evidence that diets high in sugar are associated with an increased energy content of the diet overall, which over time can lead to weight gain.

Can cutting out wheat help me lose weight?

Some people point to bread and other wheat-based foods as the main culprit for their weight gain.

Wheat is found in a wide range of foods, from bread, pasta and pizza to cereals and many other foods.

But there's not enough evidence that foods that contain wheat are any more likely to cause weight gain than any other food.

Unless you have a diagnosed health condition, such as wheat allergy, wheat sensitivity or coeliac disease, there's little evidence that cutting out wheat and other grains from your diet would benefit your health.

Grains, especially wholegrains, are an important part of a healthy, balanced diet.

Wholegrain, wholemeal and brown breads give us energy and contain B vitamins, vitamin E, fiber and a wide range of minerals.

White bread also contains an range of vitamins and minerals, but it has less fibre than wholegrain, wholemeal or brown breads.

If you prefer white bread, look for higher fibre options. Grains are also naturally low in fat.

Find out if cutting out bread could help ease bloating or other digestive symptoms.

Should people with diabetes avoid carbs?

People with diabetes should try to eat a healthy, balanced diet, as shown in the Eatwell Guide.

They should also include higher fibre starchy foods at every meal. Steer clear of cutting out entire food groups.

It's recommended that everyone with diabetes sees an registered dietitian for specific advice on their food choices. Your GP can refer you to a registered dietitian.

There's some evidence that suggests low-carbohydrate diets can lead to weight loss and improvements in blood glucose control in people with type 2 diabetes in the short term.

But it's not clear whether the diet is a safe and effective way to manage type 2 diabetes in the long term.

Weight loss from a low-carbohydrate diet may be because of a reduced intake of calories overall and not specifically as a result of eating less carbohydrate.

There also isn't enough evidence to support the use of low-carbohydrate diets in people with type 1 diabetes.

What's the role of carbohydrates in exercise?

Carbohydrates, fat and protein all provide energy, but exercising muscles rely on carbohydrates as their main source of fuel.

But muscles have limited carbohydrate stores (glycogen) and need to be topped up regularly to keep your energy up.

A diet low in carbohydrates can lead to a lack of energy during exercise, early fatigue and delayed recovery.

When is the best time to eat carbohydrates?

There's little scientific evidence that one time is better than any other.

It's recommended that you base all your meals around starchy carbohydrate foods and you try to choose higher fibre wholegrain varieties when you can.

30 DAYS KETOGENIC DIET PLAN

WEEK 1

In my eyes, simplicity is key for someone that is just starting out on an low carb diet. You don't want it to be a difficult transition (kitchen-wise), because it will be hard to just get rid of your cravings.

The first signs of ketosis are known as the "keto flu" where headaches, brain fogginess, fatigue, and the like can really rile your body up. Make sure that you're drinking plenty of waterand eating plenty of salt. The ketogenic diet is a natural diuretic and you'll be peeing more than normal. Take into account that you're peeing out electrolytes, and you can guess that you'll be having a thumping headache in no time. Keeping your salt intake and water intake high enough is very important, allowing your body to re-hydrate and re-supply your electrolytes. Doing this will help with the headaches, if not get rid of them completely.

If you need to, drink water with a sprinkling of salt in it. Just keep drinking water (I recommend 4 liters a day), and keep eating salt. It will help, trust me. If you're worried about high blood pressure and salt, don't be! Recent studies show that the sodium intake and blood pressure are not as correlated as we so once believed.

Breakfast.

For breakfast, you want to do something that's quick, easy, tasty, and of course – gives you leftovers. I suggest starting day 1 on a weekend. This way, you can make something that will last you for the entire week. The first week is all about simplicity. Nobody wants to be making breakfast before work, and we're not going to be doing that either!

Lunch.

We're also going to keep it simple here. Most of the time, it'll be salad and meat, slathered in high fat dressings and calling it a day. We don't want to get too rowdy here. You can use leftover meat from previous nights or use easy accessible canned chicken/fish. If you do use canned meats, try to read the labels and get the one that uses the least (or no) additives!

Dinner.

Dinner will be a combination of leafy greens (normally broccoli and spinach) with some meat. Again, we'll be going high on the fat and moderate on the protein.

P.S. No dessert for the first 2 weeks.

WEEK 2

Wow, week 1 is over. I hope you're still doing well on the diet and have found it pretty easy breezy to keep on track with everything!

This week we're going to be keeping is it simple for breakfast again. We're going to introduce ketoproof coffee. It's a mixture of coconut oil, butter, and heavy cream in your coffee. If this repulses you – and I know some of you are saying "WHAT?" – just put some trust in me!

This concoction is not as strange as it sounds. Butter, after all, is made out of cream. So when you blend the oil, butter, and cream together it just adds a decadent richness to your coffee that I am quite sure you'll really like!

Breakfast.

For breakfast, we are going to change it up a bit. Here's where we introduce ketoproof coffee. Now, don't get me wrong – I know some of you won't like it. If you're not an fan of coffee, then try it with tea. If you're not a fan of the taste (which is very rare), then try making a mixture of the ingredients by themselves and eating it like that. So, why ketoproof coffee?

Fat Loss. Plain and simple, the consumption of medium-chain triglycerides (MCT) has been shown to lead to greater losses in adipose tissue (fat tissue), in both animals and humans.

Fats! Do I even need to explain this one? Eating fat has been shown to lead to greater amounts of energy, more efficient energy usage, and more effective weight loss. Not to mention, it's the main component of this diet.

More Energy. Studies have shown that the rapid rate of oxidation in MCFAs (Medium Chain Fatty Acids) leads to an increase in energy expenditure. Primarily, MCFAs are converted into ketones (our best friends), are absorbed differently in the body compared to regular oils, and give us more overall energy.

Feel free to add sweetener and spices to this if you're not the biggest fan of the taste. Cinnamon, stevia, vanilla extract. Whatever you'd like to make it great tasting. You can even switch up the taste each and every day so you don't get bored!

If this is your first time drinking ketoproof coffee, I suggest taking 1-2 hours or so to drink it down. Normally when people have an large exposure to coconut oil and they're not used to it, it can make them go to the bathroom quite often. Make sure you build a tolerance to coconut oil before drinking it within a 20 minute time frame.

Lunch.

We're still keeping simple here. We can incorporate more meat from the previous night of cooking into each lunch we do. Green vegetables and high fat dressings (or vinaigrettes) are key. Making sure to balance out the fats with the amounts of protein is very important.

Dinner.

Dinner, again, will be pretty simplistic. Meats, vegetables, high fat dressings are the center of our life. Maybe even a slathering of butter on our vegetables since we're getting friskier. Don't over think things in the first 2 weeks; simple is success.

P.S. No dessert for this week either, but we'll be delving into that next week!

WEEK 3

This week we're introducing a slight fast. We're going to get full on fats in the morning and fast all the way until dinner time. Not only are there an myriad of health benefits to this, it's also easier on our eating schedule (and cooking schedule). I suggest eating (rather, drinking) your breakfast at 7am and then eating dinner at 7pm. Keeping 12 hours between your 2 meals. This will help put your body into an fasted state.

In an fasting state, our bodies can break down extra fat that's stored for the energy it needs. When we're in ketosis, our body already mimics a fasting state, being that we have little to no glucose in our bloodstream, so we use the fats in our bodies as energy.

Intermittent fasting is using the same reasoning – instead of using the fats we are eating to gain energy, we are using our stored fat. That being said, you might think it's great – you can just fast and lose more weight. You has to take into account that later on, you will need to eat extra fat in order to keep out of a starvation mode state.

There are a number of benefits shown that come from intermittent fasting. Some of these include blood lipid levels, longevity, and the much needed mental clarity.

If you find that you can't do an fast, then no big deal. Go back to week 1 and experiment as you see fit. You can eat what you want as long as it fits into your macros.

This is where things start to get more fun – less to worry about, more deliciousness to cook!

Breakfast.

We're going full on fats with breakfast, just like we did last week. This time we'll double the amount of ketoproof coffee (or tea) we drink, meaning we double the amount of coconut oil, butter, and heavy cream. It should come to quite an lot of calories, and should definitely keep us full all the way to dinner. Remember to continue drinking water like an fiend to make sure you're staying hydrated.

Lunch.

No lunch, oh no! Don't worry – the fats from the morning should keep you feeling energized and full all the way through lunch. Normally people start hitting a wall at first at around 2pm, so make sure you have plenty of water to drink, drink, and drink.

Dinner.

Well, dinner is staying the same. Meats, vegetables, and fats are almost always going to be the dinnertime norm. But don't worry – we'll mix in some bread-y type things!

And guess what, we get to eat dessert this week! Woo! We'll be creating some low carb and great tasting treats that will reward you ever so much for doing the fasting. Sweets, treats, and losing weight lucky us, right?

WEEK 4

This week we're getting stricter with our fasting. We had a full week of intermittent fasting and now we're going to skip breakfast and lunch. Water is our BEST friend here! Don't forget that you can drink coffee, tea, flavored water, and the like to get your liquids in. Keep drinking to make sure you're not thinking about your stomach. It MIGHT start growling, just ignore it – your body will adjust with time.

Now, if you're the kind of person that can't fast then you can go back and follow week 2 again. That's no big deal. Though fasting does take some time for the body to get used to, so I suggest putting your best efforts into it. Not only are the health benefits fantastic, the self-control that you gain from doing so is really a great thing.

This is by far my favorite week because it most closely resembles how I eat on a daily basis. I normally set a window of 6 hours for myself to eat in. From waking up until 5pm, I fast. After that, I am open to eating until 11pm. This is where the real fun begins. Eating copious amounts of food and being full all the way through the next day.

You get to start experimenting more with dessert and dinner. You get to snack as you please inside your window and best of all – you get to eat that protein laden chicken that you've been missing so much of!

Breakfast.

We're fasting! Black coffee if you're a caffeine addict like me. Tea, if you, are not into the coffee so much. Tea can add great health benefits like coffee also. Some of the great benefits of green tea are:

Polyphenols – These function as antioxidants in your body. The most powerful antioxidant in green tea is Epigallocatechin gallate (EGCG), which has shown to be effective against fatigue.

Improved Brain Function – Not only does green tea contain caffeine, it also contains L-theanine, which is an amino acid. L-theanine increases your GABA activity, which improves anxiety, dopamine, and alpha waves.

Increased Metabolic Rate – Green tea has been shown to improve your metabolic rate. In combination with the caffeine, this can lead up to 15% increased fat oxidization.

Lunch.

Water, water, and then some more water. You don't get to eat lunch and you don't get to eat breakfast. So make sure you keep yourself VERY hydrated. It's imperative here that you do a good job with your hydration. Remember – I recommend 4 liters a day.

Dinner.

Lots and lots of food with dessert to cover the bases! Dinner is an fantastic time for me. I suggest breaking your fast with a small snack, then after 30-45 minutes eat to your hearts content. Normally I need 2 meals to get to my macros, and I think you'll need to do the same.

WEEK 5

This is where we have to depart! Sorry to say but you're on your own. You should have plenty of leftovers that are frozen, ready, and waiting! I know an lot of you out there have trouble with timing and are busy people so making sure that some nights you make extras to freeze is important. All those leftovers you have in the freezer? Use them up! Create your own meal plan, at first using this as a guide, and then completely doing it yourself. Once you get the hang of it, it'll be a sinch – I promise you!!

IN CONCLUSION

Eating a high amount of fat, moderate protein, and low amount of carbs can have an massive impact on your health lowering your cholesterol, body weight, blood sugar, and raising your energy and mood levels.

A ketogenic diet can be hard to fathom in the beginning but isn't as hard as it's made out to be. The transition can be a little bit tough, but the growing popularity of the clean eating movement makes it easier and easier to find available low-carb foods.

Keep it straightforward and strict. You usually see better results in people who restrict their carb intake further. Try to keep your carbs as low as possible for the first month of keto. Keep it strict by cutting out excess sweets and artificial sweeteners altogether (like diet soda). Cutting these out dramatically decreases sugar cravings.

Drink water and supplement electrolytes. Most common problems come from dehydration or lack of electrolytes. When you start keto (and even in the long run), make sure that you drink plenty of water, salt your foods, and take a multivitamin. If you're still experiencing issues, you can order electrolyte supplements individually.

Track what you eat. It's so easy to over-consume on carbs when they're hidden in just about everything you pick up. Keeping track of what you eat helps control your carb intake and keep yourself accountable.